Endocrine Management of Prostatic Cancer

New Developments in Biosciences 4

Walter de Gruyter
Berlin · New York 1988

Endocrine Management of Prostatic Cancer

Editor
H. Klosterhalfen

Walter de Gruyter
Berlin · New York 1988

Editor
Prof. Dr. med. H. Klosterhalfen
Direktor der
Urologischen Klinik
Universitäts-Krankenhaus Eppendorf
Martinistraße 52
D-2000 Hamburg 20

Library of Congress Cataloging – in – Publication Data

Endocrine management of prostatic cancer / editor, H. Klosterhalfen.
p. cm. – (New development in biosciences : 4)
Proceedings of a conference held in 1987 in Hamburg.
Includes bibliographies.
ISBN 0-89925-425-X (U.S.) ; DM 48.00 (Germany ; est.)
1. Prostate – Cancer – Hormone therapy – Congresses. 2. Prostata – Cancer – Endocrine aspects – Congresses. I. Klosterhalfen, Herbert. II. Series.
[DNLM: 1. Hormones – therapeutic use – congresses. 2. Prostatic Neoplasms – drug therapy – congresses. W 3 NE 865 v. 4 / WJ 752 E 547 1987]
RC280. P7E48 1988 616.99'463061 – dc19 88 – 6945

CIP-Titelaufnahme der Deutschen Bibliothek

Endocrine management of prostatic cancer / ed.: H. Klosterhalfen. – Berlin ; New York : de Gruyter, 1988
(New developments in biosciences ; 4)
ISBN 3-11-011513-1
NE: Klosterhalfen, Herbert [Hrsg.]; GT

 Typesetting: A. Collignon, Berlin. – Printing and Binding: Elsnerdruck, Berlin. – Cover design: Rudolf Hübler. – Printed in Germany.

Contents

I Mechanism of hormonal action at cellular level and biochemistry

Mechanism and effects of androgen withdrawal therapies

N. Bruchovsky, P. S. Rennie, S. L. Goldenberg

Introduction

Until recently, androgen withdrawal therapy was restricted to a choice between bilateral orchiectomy or estrogens, usually in the form of diethylstilbestrol. When these measures failed, adrenalectomy was occasionally tried seldom yielding an objective response. The advent of antiandrogens and LHRH agonists has greatly increased the number of options, listed in table 1, which are now available for suppressing the influence of androgens on the growth of prostatic malignancy. However, the clinical indications of the various types of withdrawal therapy remain equivocal; in part this is a reflection of the multiple complex effects of

Table 1 Androgen withdrawal therapies

1. Orchiectomy
2. Diethylstilbestrol
3. Cyproterone acetate
4. Megestrol acetate
5. Flutamide
6. RU23908 (anandron)
7. LHRH agonist (buserelin, leuprolide, tryptal, zoladex)
8. Orchiectomy + cyproterone acetate
9. Orchiectomy + flutamide
10. Orchiectomy + RU23908
11. Cyproterone acetate + diethylstilbestrol
12. Megestrol acetate + diethylstilbestrol
13. LHRH agonist + diethylstilbestrol
14. LHRH agonist + cyproterone
15. LHRH agonist + cyproterone acetate + diethylstilbestrol
16. LHRH agonist + flutamide
17. LHRH agonist + RU23908
18. Ketoconazole
19. Aminoglutethimide
20. Adrenalectomy

New Developments in Biosciences 4

such treatments and the lack of information about the relative ability of each to inhibit the action of androgens in the tumour cell itself.

Mechanisms of androgen withdrawal therapy

The normal pathways of the neuro-endocrine control of gonadal function are summarized in figure 1. Testicular synthesis of testosterone accounts for 90% or more of the dihydrotestosterone formed in the prostate, the remaining being derived from weak adrenal androgens and dietary sources. Testosterone provides a negative-feedback signal to the hypothalamus regulating the secretion of LHRH and also of LH.

The principal effect of bilateral orchiectomy, as shown in figure 2, is the elimination of the testicular source of testosterone. Not only does this result in lowering of the concentration of dihydrotestosterone in the prostate but also it eliminates the negative-feedback regulation of the hypothalamus. Resultant increases in the circulating levels of LHRH and LH are probably without significance except for their association with vasomotor symptoms.

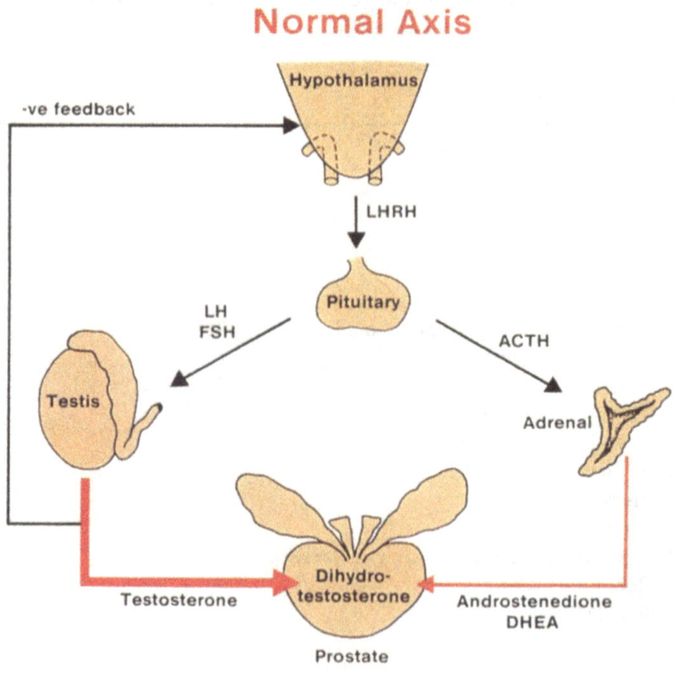

Fig. 1 Normal axis of neuro-endocrine regulation of the testis.
© N. Bruchovsky

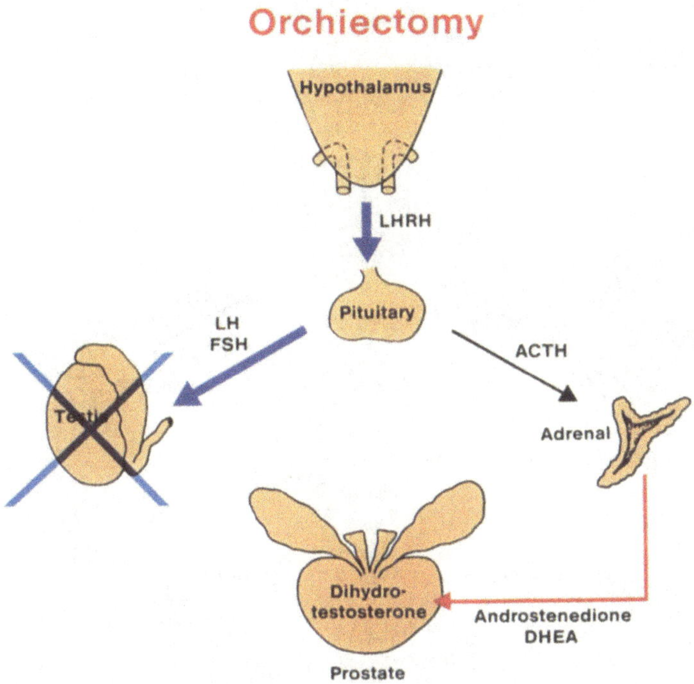

Fig. 2 Effects of orchiectomy.
© N. Bruchovsky

As depicted in figure 3, estrogenic compounds such as diethylstilbestrol override the negative-feedback inhibition of the hypothalamus by testosterone. This reduces the secretion of both LHRH and LH accompanied by marked lowering of plasma testosterone levels into the castrate range.

The action of non-steroidal antiandrogens such as flutamide and RU23908 is illustrated in figure 4. These drugs inhibit the translocation of the androgen receptor from cytoplasm to nucleus in target tissues including both the prostate and the hypothalamus. Negative-feedback signals provided by testosterone are no longer registered in the hypothalamus with resultant increases in the secretion of LHRH and LH. The testis is stimulated to increase its production of testosterone which in turn contributes to the formation of increasing amounts of dihydrotestosterone in the prostate. It is extremely doubtful that the rising titer of testosterone is wholly offset by the peripheral antiandrogenic action of flutamide and RU23908. Another consequence of the excessive production of testosterone is a higher level of estrogen in the circulation with attendant side effects such as gynecomastia.

The inhibitory action of LHRH agonists is also complex as can be seen from the schematic presented in figure 5. The pituitary is normally stimulated by the

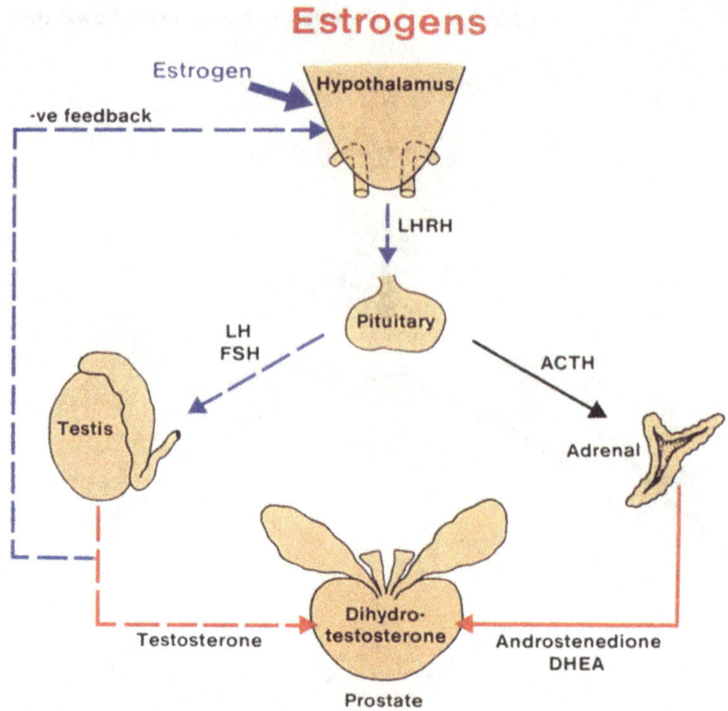

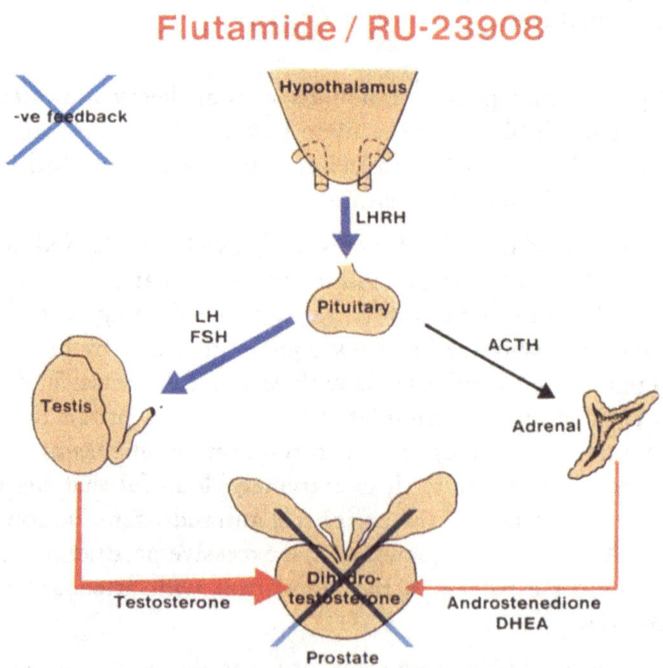

Fig. 4 Effects of flutamide and RU23908.
© N. Bruchovsky

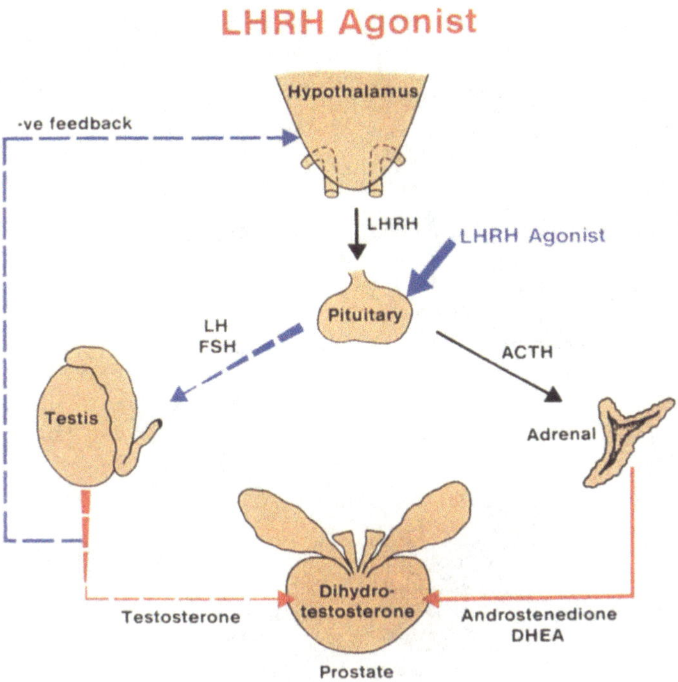

Fig. 5 Effects of LHRH agonists.
© N. Bruchovsky

pulsatile release of LHRH from the hypothalamus; when this periodicity is effaced by the continuous infusion of exogenous LHRH agonist, the pituitary becomes refractory to hypothalamic regulation. Gonadotropin secretion initially rises and then tapers off as does the secretion of testosterone by the testis. Unfortunately, the initial surge in testosterone production will sometimes result in symptoms and signs of a flare reaction.

In attempts to cancel out the adverse features of nonsteroidal antiandrogens and LHRH agonists, the agents have been combined to achieve a better balance of control of testicular function as shown diagrammatically in figure 6. On the one hand, the LHRH agonist prevents the rise in the titer of plasma testosterone caused by flutamide or RU23908 as the case may be; on the other hand, either of the latter two agents (or other antiandrogens ie. cyproterone acetate) reduce the risk of a flare reaction that may occur during the surge in the concentration of plasma testosterone caused by the LHRH agonist. Although it has been hypothesized that the effects of weak androgens originating in the adrenal glands will be counteracted by antiandrogenic medication, available evidence indicates that adrenal androgens have no effect on the growth of the prostate [2]. The

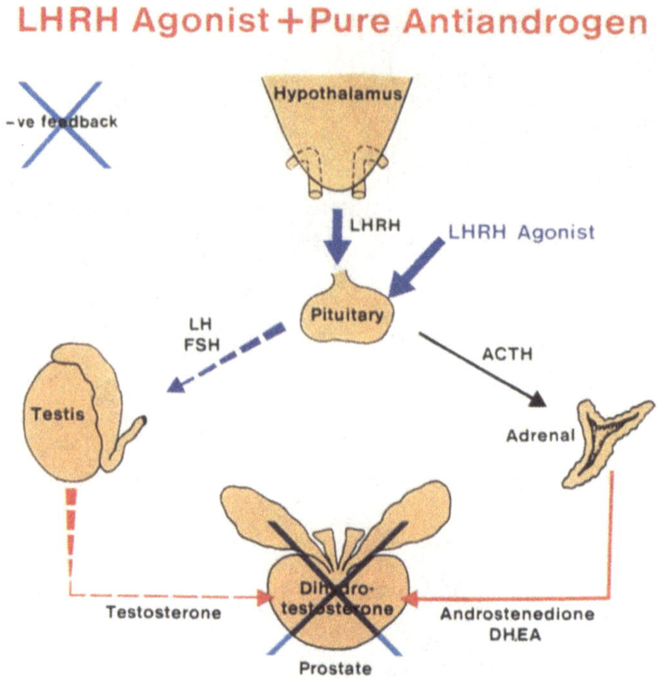

Fig. 6 Effects of LHRH agonist combined with a non-steroidal (pure) antiandrogen. © N. Bruchovsky

only justification for combining an antiandrogen with an LHRH agonist would be to avert the untoward side-effects associated with a flare reaction.

Progestational antiandrogens such as cyproterone acetate and megestrol acetate are equivalent to the combination of an LHRH agonist and a non-steroidal antiandrogen since they both act centrally to inhibit the secretion of LHRH by the hypothalamus and peripherally to interfere with the receptor mechanism. Details of the mode of action are given in figure 7. In the example shown, cyproterone acetate, owing to its progestational activity, overrides the negative-feedback inhibition of the hypothalamus by testosterone; in addition, it is active peripherally in prostatic tissue where it reduces the concentration of nuclear androgen receptor. This type of therapy is much easier to administer than the facsimile described in figure 6, and is well tolerated by patients, but requires reinforcement with low-dose diethylstilbestrol (0.1 mg) if maintenance of plasma testosterone in the castrate range is essential. In fact, the combination of cyproterone acetate and low-dose diethylstilbestrol, or alternatively, megestrol acetate and low-dose diethylstilbestrol, appears to be one of the most potent forms of androgen withdrawal therapy presently available.

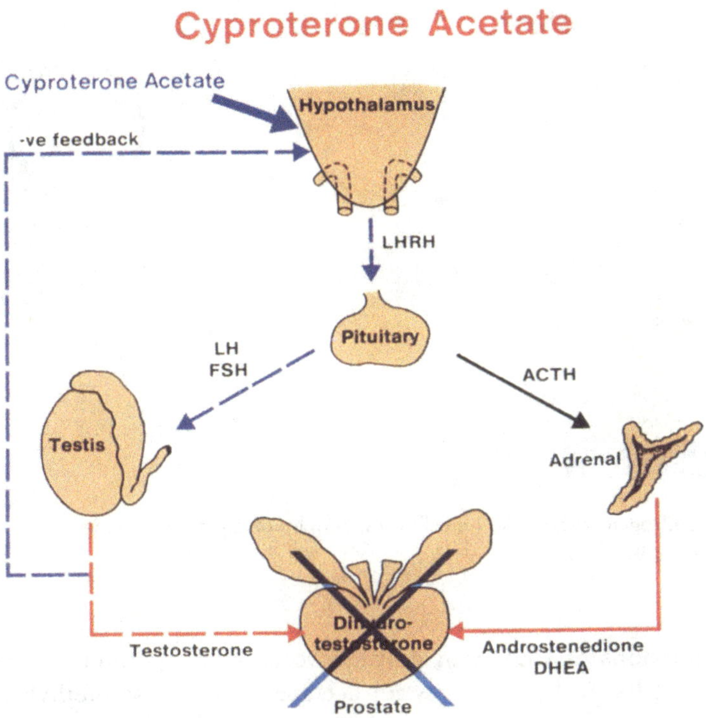

Fig. 7 Effects of cyproterone acetate.
© N. Bruchovsky

Relative effectiveness of alternative androgen withdrawal therapies

Since the earliest detectable effects of androgen withdrawal therapy consist of a drop in the whole tissue and nuclear concentrations of dihydrotestosterone, and the discharge of nuclear androgen receptor into the cytoplasm, such end-points can be used to compare the effectiveness of different withdrawal regimens after a relatively short course of treatment [4]. In rat prostate the redistribution of androgenic markers is maximal on the third day after castration when no appreciable change in volume has yet taken place but the tissue is poised to involute. The change in whole-tissue concentration of dihydrotestosterone produced by bilateral orchiectomy is an index of this type which may be compared to the effects of several alternative androgen withdrawal therapies; results of such an analysis are summarized in table 2.

From a normal level of 14.2 ± 1.3 pmol/mg DNA (mean ± SE), the whole-tissue concentration of dihydrotestosterone declines to 5% of normal following surgical

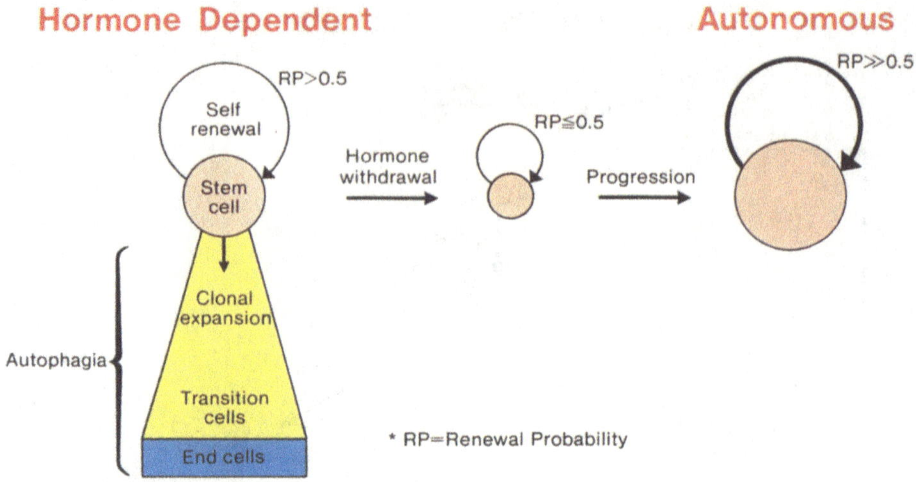

Fig. 8 Effects of androgen withdrawal on cellular hierarchy of prostatic tumours. © N. Bruchovsky

castration. Reductions of similar magnitude occur with cyproterone acetate + low-dose diethylstilbestrol and megestrol acetate + low-dose diethylstilbestrol; the changes are highly significant ($p < 0.001$). Similarly, significant ($p < 0.05$) but less pronounced reductions are produced by leuprolide + flutamide, low-dose diethylstilbestrol and megestrol acetate. The remaining treatments forming Group III fail to produce significant results. When administered as single agents, cyproterone acetate, megestrol acetate and low-dose diethylstilbestrol are markedly less active than the estrogen-antiandrogen combinations. The difference in activity is in keeping with the synergism between progestational and estrogenic compounds in suppressing pituitary gonadotropin. Since none of the alternative androgen withdrawal therapies containing an antiandrogen is more effective than surgical castration in initiating early tissue involution, the inhibition of adrenal androgens does not add to the effects of testicular ablation. The observations also indicate that the most potent androgen withdrawal therapies, cyproterone acetate + low-dose diethylstilbestrol and megestrol acetate + low-dose diethylstilbestrol, at best approximate but do not surpass the acute results of bilateral orchiectomy.

Clinical effects of androgen withdrawal therapy

Owing to the evidence of marked synergistic activity between low-dose diethylstilbestrol and cyproterone acetate, this combination was tested in a pilot study at our institution for activity against Stage D2 prostatic carcinoma [3]. Associated with a rapid decline in the concentration of serum testosterone, there was a high initial response rate as judged on the basis of NPCP criteria; this evidence and other details are summarized in table 2.

In the group of 51 patients entered into the study, complete and partial responses were observed in 42 and the disease was stabilized in another 8 yielding an overall objective response rate of 98%. In 49 patients there was a measurable abnormality of either the prostatic component of the disease or in other soft tissue sites, chiefly lymph nodes. The tumour regressed in 41 of these cases and in another 8 growth was temporarily arrested. In contrast, only 13 complete and partial responses were seen in the 47 patients with abnormal bone scans at the initiation of therapy; the skeletal disease was at best only stabilized in the majority of patients. These observations clearly demonstrate how potent androgen withdrawal therapy results in good control of soft tissue disease but is far less effective

Table 2 Effects of androgen withdrawal therapies on the concentrations of whole-tissue dihydrotestosterone*

p (t-test)	Treatments	Percent of intact control
Group I $p < 0.001$	Castration	5.0
	Cyproterone acetate + DES**	4.4
	Megestrol acetate + DES	6.5
Group II $p < 0.05$	Leuprolide + flutamide	26.9
	DES	44.1
	Megestrol acetate	50.5
Group III Not significant	Leuprolide + cyproterone acetate + DES	50.4
	Cyproterone acetate	64.3
	Leuprolide	69.7
	Leuprolide + cyproterone acetate	83.3
	Leuprolide + RU23908	87.4
	Flutamide	113.9
	RU23908	124.6

* Groups of 5–7 rats were injected s. c. on days 1, 2, and 3 with the agents shown at doses equivalent to those used clinically except for diethylstilbestrol which was administered at a 10-fold lower dose. The non-castrated control group and the castrated control group each received injections of vehicle alone. On the 4th experimental day the animals were sacrificed. Whole-tissue homogenates prepared from the pooled ventral prostates were assayed by radioimmunoassay for dihydrotestosterone. The mean result for each treatment (average from 5–34 experiments) is expressed as a percentage of the control mean (100%).

** diethylstilbestrol

Table 3 Response to cyproterone acetate + low-dose diethylstilbestrol

	Overall	Prostate and soft tissue	Bone scan
Abnormal before treatment	51 (100%)	49 (100%)	48 (100%)
Complete and partial responses	42 (82%)	41 (84%)	13 (27%)
Stable disease	8 (16%)	8 (16%)	29 (60%)
No response	1 (2%)	0 (0%)	6 (13%)
Progression within 2 years*	26 (52%)	6 (12%)	22 (44%)

* in group of 50 responders

against skeletal metastases which are relatively resistant to the withdrawal of androgens. The failure of treatment to adequately control skeletal metastases is also evident from the data in table 3; in the group of 26 patients who progressed within 2 years, the skeletal disease became worse in 22 as revealed by bone scan whereas the prostate and soft tissue malignancy showed measurable advance in only 6. This dissociation between the responsiveness of carcinoma in the prostate and lymph nodes as compared to that in bone implies that skeletal metastases represent a very different form of prostatic malignancy as compared with the primary tumour.

Despite the objective response rate of 98%, no major gains in survival were observed with 82% of the patients surviving 1 year and 47%, 2 years; the median survival time was 23.5 months. Hence, even with a very potent form of androgen withdrawal therapy, the lethal component of the disease will not be eliminated.

Limitations of androgen withdrawal therapy

It is a misconception that the benefits of androgen withdrawal therapy can be improved by resorting to more radical forms of androgen deprivation. Such therapy has limitations and in the extreme is potentially harmful. Several of the shortcomings inherent in this approach are obvious from the adverse biological changes which take place in the Shionogi carcinoma as it progresses from an androgen-dependent to an androgen-independent state. In male mice, the transplantable parent tumour grows with a doubling time of about 24 hours and upon castration of the host animal regresses almost completely in 7 to 10 days. After a subclinical phase lasting 20 to 30 days when the tumour is either very small or not palpable, recurrent growth is detected and is characterized by slightly longer doubling time. Unlike the parent cells, the recurrent tumour does not respond to further androgen withdrawal therapy.

A limiting dilution assay was developed in our laboratory to measure the stem cell content of the parent and recurrent tumours. The analysis was done by injecting a decreasing number of parent of recurrent tumour cells into several groups of male animals and noting the incidence of tumour takes in each group. At the point where this falls off to 50%, there is on average 1 clonogenic cell per inoculum. Since the number of tumour cells in the latter is known, an estimate is obtained of the proportion of stem cells in the overall population of tumour cells.

In applying this analysis to the Shionogi carcinoma before and after castration, we found that there is one stem cell per 6000 tumour cells in the parent tumour compared with 1 stem cell per 200 tumour cells in the recurrent tumour. Therefore, the effect of androgen withdrawal therapy is to cause a mark 30-fold enrichment of stem cells in the recurrent malignancy.

Such results are consistent with the model shown in fig. 8 (p. 10) which has been discussed in detail elsewhere [1]. A hormone-dependent tumour may be thought of as being a functional hierarchy of stem cells and differentiated daughter cells which through clonal expansion form the bulk of the malignancy. Androgen withdrawal may bring about a large reduction in tumour volume but for the most part this involves the selective elimination of the non-stem daughter cells via the expression of an autophagic process. Any differentiation of stem cells that takes place after androgen-withdrawal would not be associated with the induction of the cytolytic (autophagic) mechanism responsible for cell death; for practical purposes the androgen-dependent cells are permanently lost from the tumour.

The fate of stem cells following androgen-withdrawal is somewhat ambiguous. In the Shionogi carcinoma, the number of stem cells decreases by approximately 2 logarithms in an androgen-poor environment; this suggests that any castration-like treatment will have a significant impact on the size of the stem-cell compartment. However, the surviving stem cells continue to multiply giving rise to a recurrent tumour with a greatly augmented pool of stem cells. It would appear that the stem cells increase their relative proportions owing in part to the absence of any androgen-induced differentiation. Until proven otherwise, it should be assumed that the risk of metastasis may be increased in a tumour with an enriched non-differentiated stem-cell population [1]. Of more immediate concern, however, is the possibility that potent androgen withdrawal therapies by accentuating this whole process actually jeopardize the outcome of hormonal treatment in the longer term.

Conclusions

The key points reviewed in this report may be summarized as follows: first, none of the alternative androgen withdrawal therapies are more effective than surgical castration; second, castration is best approximated by the combinations of cyproterone acetate + low-dose diethylstilbestrol and megestrol acetate + low-dose diethylstilbestrol; third, the inhibition of adrenal androgens by antiandrogenic agents does not add to the effects of testicular ablation; fourth, androgen withdrawal therapy is limited by the relative resistance of skeletal metastases; lastly, such therapy is also conducive to the outgrowth of androgen-independent stem cells.

Acknowledgments

Our research is supported by grants from the National Cancer Institute of Canada, and the Medical Research Council of Canada. The artistic work was designed and prepared by Pauly Wong of the Graphics Division of the University of Alberta. We thank Cynthia Wells for typing the manuscript.

References

[1] Bruchovsky, N., E. M. Brown, E. M. Coppin et al.: The endocrinology and treatment of prostate toumor progression. In: D. S. Coffey, N. Bruchovsky, W. A. Gardner, Jr. et al. (eds.): Current Concepts and Approaches to the Study of Prostate Cancer, pp. 347–387. Alan R. Liss, New York 1987.

[2] Coffey, D. S., K. J. Pienta: New concepts in studying the control of normal and cancer growth of the prostate. In: Coffey, D. S., N. Bruchovsky, W. A. Gardner, Jr. et al. (eds.): Current Concepts and Approaches to the Study of Prostate Cancer, pp. 1–73. Alan R. Liss, New York 1987.

[3] Goldenberg, S. L., N. Bruchovsky, P. S. Rennie et al.: The combination of cyproterone acetate and low-dose diethylstilbestrol in the treatment of advanced prostatic carcinoma. Submitted for publication.

[4] Rennie, P. S., N. Bruchovsky, S. L. Goldenberg et al.: Relative effectiveness of alternative androgen withdrawal therapies in initiating regression of rat prostate. Submitted for publication.

Target-cell response to androgen withdrawal

K. D. Voigt, H. Klein

The weight loss of the prostate after androgen withdrawal by surgical or chemical castration is a well-known phenomenon. For the rat prostate, the first quantitative description of the accompanying decrease in cell number have been published by Bruchovsky and co-workers several years ago [6]. They observed a plateau during the first 3 days followed by a steep fall in cell number until the 7th or 8th day post-castration. Subsequent androgen replacement resulted in an increase in cell number to the original level within the next 6 to 7 days, demonstrating the preserved capacity of surviving cells to restore the original organ structure. This paper will concentrate on events occuring during the first phases of prostatic response, that is during the plateau and the subsequent period of involution.

Summarizing our data about cellular macromolecules during the post-castration time course, the weight and protein loss as well as the decrease in RNA and DNA content of the prostate at first glance appeared to occur in parallel. However, a closer examination revealed differences: The DNA curve was generally flatter, and the DNA was the only parameter having a plateau over the first 2 days, while the other parameters showed plateaus over only 1 or 1.5 days. Considering the morphology of single cells as measured by morphometrical techniques, a shrinkage of the cellular volume also occured after a latency period of 2 days. The more rapid decrease in prostatic RNA content as compared to the DNA correlated with this cell shrinkage.

Considering the number of prostatic cells, English and co-workers have reported that androgen withdrawal results in a drop in epithelial cell number of approximately 90% within 7 days, while the corresponding decrease in the stromal cells was approximately 70% [3]. To our knowledge, the exact time course of the fall in cell number in the prostatic epithelium and stroma after androgen withdrawal has not been previously described. We have investigated the number of prostatic cells using morphometrical techniques and found that the stromal cell number decreased constantly but more slowly, and even after 14 days had not reached this level reported by others. In contrast, the epithelial cells decreased rapidly until the 8th day post-castration at which time the cell number was reduced by approximately 2/3. The plateau formed during the first two days was not so well defined as expected from the DNA values. When the loss of cells and the shrinkage of surviving epithelial cells are considered together, the prostatic weight loss would be expected to be in the order of 75 – 80%. The actual weight loss observed in our experiments was approximately 80%, confirming the results of these morphometric studies.

New Developments in Biosciences 4

Obviously and in agreement with English and co-workers, androgen withdrawal mainly affects the epithelial cell population. Two questions are raised by these observations concerning on one hand the exact duration and significance of the plateau, and on the other hand the fate of the lost epithelial cells.

In histological pictures of the prostate taken at varying times post-castration, both the shrinking of epithelial cells as well as their death are observable: Under physiological stimulation by androgen, the tall cylindrical epithelium of the prostate reflects the high secretory activity. 14 days after castration, the glandular ducts appear as flat layers of involuted epithelial cells expressing the shrinkage of surviving cells during the post-castration period. Morphological correlates of the loss of cells are apparent as apoptotic bodies within the epithelium, which are remains of dead epithelial cells. Apoptosis is a physiological form of cell death distinct from necrosis. Biochemical mechanisms underlying the process of apoptosis have been the focus of much interest during the past few years. For the rat prostate, apoptosis was first described by Kerr and Searle in 1973 on the basis of light- and electron-microscopy [5]. According to these authors, apoptotic bodies are finally eliminated from the tissue by expulsion into the glandular lumen.

A systematic examination of histological preparations gave the impression of a correlation between the duration of androgen withdrawal and the frequency of apoptotic cell death. Therefore, we have morphologically quantitated the number of intraepithelial apoptotic bodies in histological sections of prostates taken at varying points of time after castration and have extrapolated these values on total organ volumes:

Even under physiological hormonal stimulation, low numbers of approximately 3000 apoptotic bodies per organ are detectable. Following androgen withdrawal, the number of apoptotic bodies remains at this level for at least 30 hours. After this period, a rapid and massive increase in the frequency of apoptosis in the organ was recorded. By 33 hours post-castration, the number of apoptotic bodies per organ had doubled, and by 48 hours had increased by 50-fold. During the next 24 hours, the degree of apoptosis remained at this maximum level and then began to decline after 72 hours with approximately the same kinetics as the increase approaching the starting line between the 7th and 8th day post-castration. *Qualitatively*, the course of the apoptosis curve reflects the epithelial cell loss in this phase. *Quantitatively*, the number of apoptotic bodies at one point of time on the one hand and the epithelial cell loss per day on the other hand differed by 2 orders of magnitude. This discrepancy points to a rapid onset of apoptosis after the latency period and to a rapid elimination of the apoptotic bodies from the tissue.

Approximately 1/3 of the originally existing epithelial cells are spared after the massive apoptotic cell death ending one week after the initiation of androgen withdrawal. At least 3 hypotheses can be proposed to clarify this phenomenon:

1. The prostate contains different epithelial cell clones, a portion of which exists and grow independently of androgens, comprising the surviving fraction.
2. Prostatic epithelial cells adapt under the condition of androgen withdrawal according to statistically probability. The surviving cells which have undergone this adaptation form the epithelium of the involuted prostate.
3. Androgen requirement of prostatic epithelial cells depends on functional state and/or phase in the cell cycle. Also in this case the survival of epithelial cells does not require the assumption of different cell clones. At present, our preliminary data point in the direction of the last hypotheses.

Prostatic target cell responses to the withdrawal of androgenic stimulation are not restricted to morphologically visible processes, but they also affect specific functions of the surviving cells including steroid metabolism and the androgen receptor system. Steroids, steroid receptors, and the enzymes 5α-reductase, 17β-hydroxysteroid oxidoreductase (17β-HSOR), and 3αβ-hydroxysteroid oxidoreductase (3αβ-HSOR) were quantitated in the tissue and subcellular fractions according to standard methods previously described [1, 2,4].

Monitoring the time course of enzyme activities post-castration, decreases in 5α-reductase as well as 17β-HSOR beginning on the first day were observed. In contrast, alterations in the activity of 3αβ-HSOR were insignificant during the first week. These results suggest that the syntheses of 5α-reductase and of 17β-HSOR are androgen-dependent while the synthesis of 3αβ-HSOR does not appear to depend on androgens. In order to test this hypothesis, we have performed restimulation experiments at varying time points during the course of androgen withdrawal. For this purpose, testosterone containing silicon capsules were implanted subcutaneously into rats to restore physiological testosterone levels, and the prostates were sampled 20 hours later: As compared to values in androgen-depleted, untreated animals, activities of 5α-reductase and 17β-HSOR were massively increased by this treatment supporting the hypothesis of androgen dependence of these enzymes. Furthermore, the failure to observe an alteration in the 3αβ-HSOR activity during these restimulation experiments also supports the contention that this enzyme is androgen-independent, at least following short-term hormonal manipulations. The possible biological implication of these results is underlined by ratio of 5α-reductase to 3αβ-HSOR, reflecting the process of formation to inactivation of DHT. Under the conditions of the restimulation experiments, this ratio lies clearly over the starting levels under physiological conditions, further favoring the formation of DHT.

A parallel inspection of the androgen receptor content and distribution clarifies two events: 1. Androgen withdrawal leads to a quick and pronounced decrease of nuclear receptor content and 2. androgen replacement induces a very rapid and significant translocation of receptor protein into nuclear structures, the total increase in receptor content being mainly due to this process. Remarkably, the nuclear receptor concentration assayed after androgenic restimulation of androgen-deprived animals was found to exceed values measured under physiological conditions.

The consequence of both phenomena i. e. increase in DHT synthesis and in nuclear receptor content should be an augmentation of nuclear DHT. In fact, nuclear DHT levels observed under the condition of restimulation experiments, exceeded the physiological concentrations. Furthermore, the ratio of DHT to 3α-androstanediol was approximately doubled in comparison to the physiological starting level. This should allow a quick and substantial biological reaction of the target cells to restored androgenic stimulation.

In conclusion, the castration induced involution of the rat prostate involves mainly the epithelial compartment. The involution of the epithelium is the consequence of the death of approximately 2/3 of the epithelial cells with a concurrent shrinking of the surviving cell fraction. Cell death appearing as apoptosis occurs after a latency period of at least 30 hours following androgen withdrawal and thereafter proceeds rapidly. Under these conditions, the prostatic androgen metabolism do not switch in a way to balance the decreased formation of DHT by a reduced inactivation rate. On the contrary, the sinking of the 5α-reductase/3αβ-HSOR ratio leads to androgen depletion of the tissue. Prostatic androgen metabolism, however, responds rapidly to replacement of androgens favoring the accumulation of DHT.

References

[1] Bartsch, W., C. Knabbe, K. D. Voigt: Regulation and compartimentalization of androgens in rat prostate and muscle. J. steroid. Biochem. **19** (1983) 929 – 937.

[2] Braun, B. E., M. Krieg: Sexual activity influences organ weight and androgen metabolism of rat prostate, bulbocavernosus/levator ani muscle and kidney. J. steroid. Biochem. **19** (1983) 1763 – 1768.

[3] English, H. F., J. R. Drago, R. J. Santen: Cellular response to androgen depletion and repletion in the rat ventral prostate: Autoradiography and morphometric analysis. Prostate 7 (1985) 41 – 51.

[4] Huang, J. K., W. Bartsch, K. D. Voigt: Interactions of an anti-androgen (cyproterone acetate) with the androgen receptor system and its biological action in the rat ventral prostate. Acta endocrinol. (Copenh.) **109** (1985) 569 – 576.

[5] Kerr, J. F. R., J. Searle: Deletion of cells by apoptosis during castration-induced involution of the rat prostate. Virchows Archiv B. Zellpathol. **13** (1973) 87 – 102.

[6] Lesser, B., N. Bruchovsky: The effects of testosterone, 5α-dihydrotestosterone and adenosine 3'5'-monophosphate on cell proliferation and differentiation in the rat prostate. Biochim. Biophys. Acta **308** (1973) 426 – 427.

Effects of chronic treatment with an LH-RH agonist on human testis tissue

I. T. Huhtaniemi

Introduction

Luteinizing hormone-releasing hormone (LH-RH) agonist analogues are today an established alternative for hormonal treatment of prostatic carcinoma [3, 15, 20, 22, 24]. The paradoxic inhibitory effects of the peptide result in inhibition of pituitary gonadotropin secretion and testicular androgen production. This chemical form of castration decreases circulating testosterone to levels indistinguishable from those after surgical orchiectomy which is the basis for equal therapeutic effects of both treatment modalities.

The inhibition of testicular androgen production by LH-RH agonists is now well established [3, 17, 20, 22, 24], but the exact mechanism of this action is still poorly understood in the human. Although the pituitary and gonadal suppression by LH-RH and its analogues has been widely examined in laboratory animals (especially rodents), the results are applicable to the human only to a limited extent due to clearcut species differences [4, 10, 20].

Since the therapeutic effect of LH-RH agonists is clear in prostatic cancer, exact insight into their mechanism of action in testicular suppression is not crucial from the clinical point of view. However, if the same peptides are to be used for other clinical indications, especially for male contraception, it will be important to know in details the mechanisms of the LH-RH agonist induced pituitary-testicular suppression. For this reason, we examined the direct testicular effects of chronic LH-RH agonist therapy in a group of prostatic cancer patients.

Materials and methods

Seven patients (age 58 – 79 yr) with advanced prostatic cancer, confirmed by biopsy, were treated for 6 months with a potent LH-RH agonist analogue (buserelin, Hoechst, 600 μg 3 times daily) [15 – 17]. All patients were recently diagnosed and had not received any previous treatment for prostatic cancer. Consent

New Developments in Biosciences 4

was obtained after the therapeutic options available were explained. Buserelin treatment was offered for 6 months after which the patients underwent surgical castration as continuation of endocrine therapy. The testis tissue obtained from these patients was used for the studies.

Another group (n = 10) of age-matched patients with similar stage of the disease served as controls. These patients were orchiectomized as the first form of treatment, and the testis tissue obtained from them served as control tissue.

The testis tissue obtained was used for the following measurements: endogenous levels of testosterone and receptors for LH and FSH, basal and gonadotropin-stimulated production by testis tissue slices of testosterone, some of its precursor steroids and cyclic AMP. Tissue samples were also analyzed by light and electron microscopy. The quality of spermatogenesis was evaluated by the score count method Johnsen [19]. Scores of 1–10, corresponding to the histological findings were given. In short, 1 indicated the presence of no cells in tubular sections, and 10 indicated complete spermatogenesis. Details of the experimental and analytical procedures are available in the original reports on these studies [15–17]. In addition to the testicular measurements, circulating hormone parameters of the patients were followed closely, both before and during the peptide treatment and after orchiectomy [15, 17].

Results

Biochemical findings

The testosterone concentration of control testis tissues was 1.40 ± 0.21 nmol/g wet weight (± SE, n = 10). A decrease of 95%, to 0.072 ± 0.013 nmol/g ($p < 0.01$, n = 7), was observed in testes obtained after 6 months of buserelin treatment (fig. 1). Interestingly, the LH receptor level was unaffected by the treatment, but the high affinity binding of FSH decreased by about 60% (fig. 1). The low-affinity population of FSH receptors showed more variable response to the gonadotropin suppression [15].

In vitro production of cyclic AMP by testicular slices was similar in both groups of tissues, with only marginal (20–30%) stimulation by hCG (tab. 1). In contrast, the testosterone production was decreased by about 95% (tab. 1). The low stimulability of this parameter by hCG (39–45%) was also maintained during buserelin treatment. In addition to testosterone, the incubation media were analyzed for some of its steroidal precursors and the metabolite 5α-dihydrotestosterone (fig. 2). The total production rate of the steroids measured was decreased by 73% in the buserelin treatment group: controls 3170 ±570 pmol/g tissue (± SE, n = 5), after buserelin treatment 870 ± 180 pmol/g tissue (n = 4)

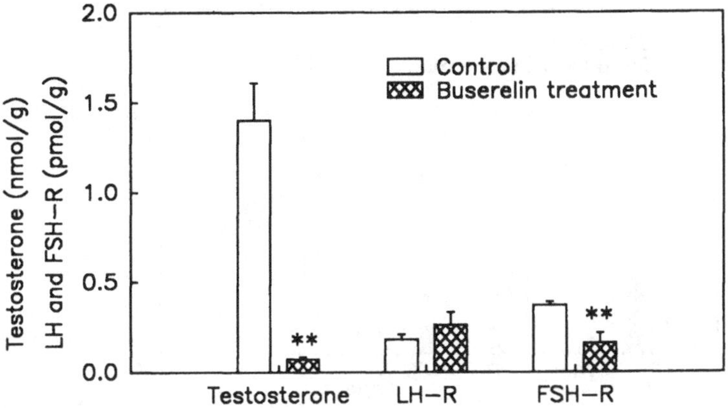

Fig. 1 Testicular testosterone, and LH- and FHS-receptors in tissue obtained from control (n = 10) and buserelin treated (n = 7) patients (mean ± SE) (ref. 17). The asterisks indicate significant difference between the control and buserelin treatment groups (**, $p < 0.01$).

Table 1 Production of cAMP and testosterone (T) by slices of testis tissue from the control and buserelin treated patients. Both the basal and hCG stimulated (300 ng/ml) rates of production were measured [17].

	Control (n = 7)	Buserelin (n = 7)
cAMP production (pmol/g tissue)		
Basal	157 ± 36	171 ± 35
hCG-stimulation (% increase of basal level)	23 ± 6.7	16 ± 7.7
T production (pmol/g tissue)		
Basal	2.17 ± 0.42	0.12 ± 0.033**
hCG-stimulation (% increase of basal level)	45 ± 12	39 ± 16

** $p < 0.01$ vs. control

($p < 0.01$). Production rates of pregnenolone, progesterone and dehydroepiandrosterone were not significantly affected by the treatment, whereas the formation of the other steroids, 17-hydroxyprogesterone, androstenedione, testosterone and 5α-dihydrotestosterone, decreased 71–90% ($p < 0.01 - 0.05$).

Morphological studies

Testis weights were similar in both groups of patients (tab. 2). The Johnsen scores [19] of spermatogenesis were considerably reduced, with highly variable

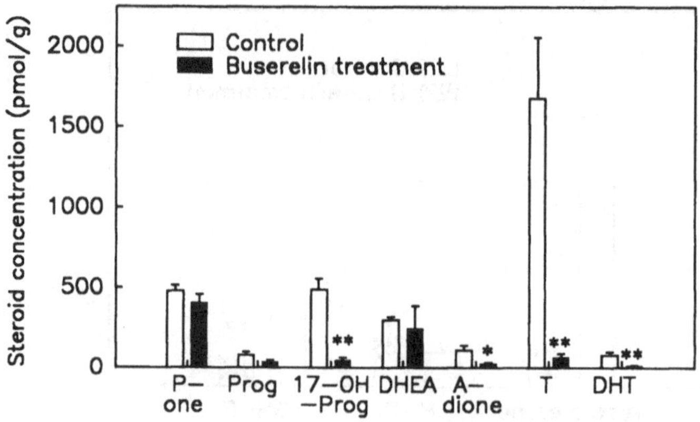

Fig. 2 Production of pregnenolone (P-one), progesterone (Prog), 17-hydroxyprogesterone (17-OH-Prog), dehydroepiandrosterone (DHEA), androstenedione (A-dione), testosterone (T) and 5α-dihydrotestosterone (DHT) by slices of human testis tissue from control (n = 5) and buserelin treated (n = 4) patients in vitro (ref. 15, 17). The concentrations presented indicate steroid produced per g tissue (mean ± SE) during a 3-h incubation period. The asterisks indicate differences in the production rates between the control and buserelin treatment groups (*, $p < 0.05$; **, $p < 0.01$).

Table 2 Weights and histological data on testis tissue of the control and buserelin treated patients (mean ± SE) [17]

	Control (n = 14)	Buserelin (n = 7)
Testis weight (g)	9.64 ± 1.01	8.56 ± 1.18
Johnsen score	5.57 ± 0.62	3.36 ± 0.88*
Leydig cells/cm³ tissue (× 10⁶)	27.5 ± 3.75	33.4 ± 7.30
Sertoli cells/cm³ (× 10⁶)	13.3 ± 3.57	12.6 ± 4.18
Tubular diameter (um)	145 ± 5.2	127 ± 4.1*

* $p < 0.05$ vs. control

range (1.5 – 8), already in the control patients (5.57 ± 0.62). A slight decrease to 3.36 ± 0.88 ($p < 0.05$) was observed during buserelin treatment, but again, the variability of the scores was great (range 1 – 8). No differences were found between the two groups in the numbers of Leydig and Sertoli cells, either expressed per unit weight of tissue or per whole testis. However, the tubular diameters were slightly lower ($p < 0.05$) in testes of the buserelin treated patients (tab. 2).

Most of the control patients (fig. 3) showed seminiferous tubuli with all types of germ cells present. However, none of them showed fully normal seminiferous

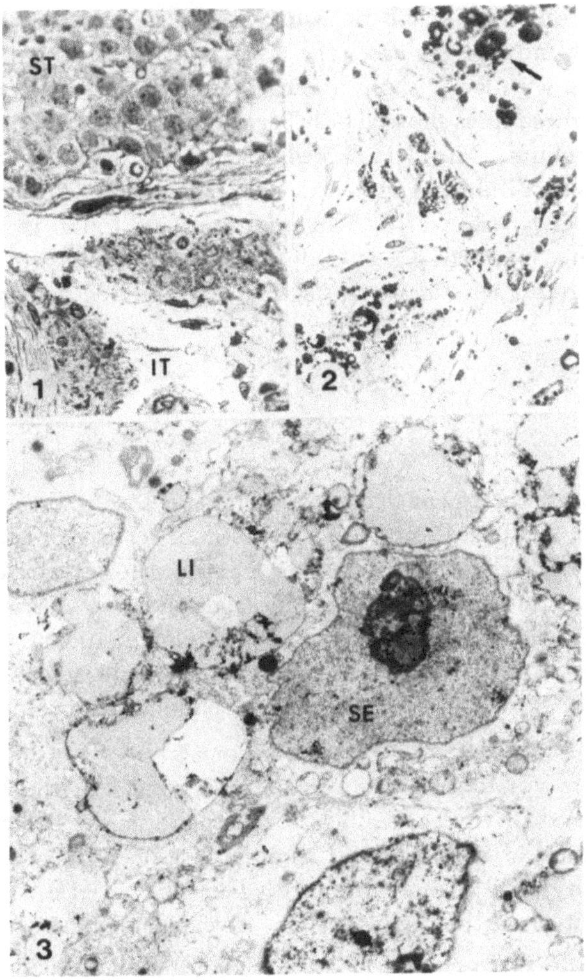

Fig. 3 Light micrograph of a toluidine-blue stained semi-thin section of a control testis (Johnsen score 8). All types of germ cells are present in the seminiferous tubules (ST) and the Leydig cells in the interstitial tissue (IT) are normal. Magnification 520 × (1); light micrograph of the testis from a patient treated with buserelin (Johnsen score 2–3). The seminiferous epithelium contains only a few cells and there are vast lipid accumulations (arrow). The Leydig cells also appear dedifferentiated. Magnification 520 × (2); electron micrograph of the seminiferous epithelium of a patient (Johnsen score 1.5) treated with buserelin. Sertoli cells (SE) contain large lipid droplets (LI). Magnification 7800 × (ref. 14) (3).

epithelium, probably due to the high age and health condition. The maximum Johnsen scrore was 8 indicating that the best spermatogenesis found in this material included only a limited number of elongated spermatids in the seminiferous epithelium. The Leydig cells showed in electron microscopy features of poorly stimulated condition.

In the buserelin treated group (fig. 3), all patients showed disturbances of the seminiferous epithelium. In most severe cases the normal structure of testis was replaced by fibrous tissue with only slight indication of preservation of the tubular structure. Most of these cases showed only Sertoli cells and spermatogonia in the seminiferous epithelium. The Sertoli cells contained typically greatly enhanced amounts of fagocytozed lipid material, and the basement membrane was frequently thickened. Clear signs of dedifferentiation were found in Leydig cells of all samples from the treatment group. However, it should be emphasized that the suppression of spermatogenesis was variable also in the treatment group.

Discussion

Although the LH-RH agonist treatment decreases peripheral serum testosterone to the castrate range [3, 15, 20, 22, 24], possible low residual activity of the testis tissue cannot be excluded by periferal serum measurements only. Our data clearly show that only 5% of the endogenous testosterone level and testosterone production of the testis tissue remains after long term buserelin treatment. Effects on the prostate of such low androgen levels (plus the adrenal androgens) cannot be totally excluded [1, 20]. However, the necessity of elimination of such low remaining androgen levels [20] is still open.

The low response to acute gonadotropin stimulation is typical of the human testis tissue both in vivo and in vitro [11, 23]. In spite of the clear decrease of testosterone production, the LH receptors and stimulability of cyclic AMP and testosterone production by hCG were maintained. The lack of effect on LH receptors could mean that these binding sites are not dependent on normal circulating levels of gonadotropins. In fact, it has been shown in animal experiments that maintenance LH receptors is dependent on prolactin and not on LH [12, 18]. It was important to note that the testis tissue maintains its capability of responding with increased androgen production to gonadotropic stimulation. This emphasizes the necessity of total and persistent gonadotropin suppression during the therapy.

The behaviour of the LH and the high affinity FSH receptors was different; only the latter receptor sites decrease by about 50% during buserelin treatment. Therefore, the FSH receptors are either intimately dependent on normal circulating gonadotropin levels (LH and/or FSH), or indirectly on normal Leydig cell function (intratesticular androgen level).

Analysis of testosterone precursor formation revealed that the steroidogenesis was not completely blocked during the 6 month buserelin treatment. In fact, the production rates of pregnenolone, progesterone and DHEA were not affected at all. Clear decreases occurred only in steroids beyond the 3β-hydroxysteroid dehydrogenase step, suggesting that particularly this enzyme is affected during the peptide treatment.

Although the cessation of androgen production was a constant finding, the impairment of spermatogenesis, as monitored by tubular histology, was variable. Decreased gonatotropin levels [15, 17] and a 95% drop in intratesticular testosterone were therefore not sufficient to stop completely spermatogenesis. Similar inconsistency of spermatogenic effect has been found in studies on the applicability of LH-RH agonists for male contraception [2, 7, 21]. Since both gonadotropin action and high intratesticular testosterone are required for spermatogenesis, the failure of the LH-RH agonist effect appears surprising. The following explanations could be speculated: Firstly, the testosterone concentration of normal human testis tissue is extremely high, up to 10-fold higher than in several other mammalian spieces [5, 6, 9]. Therefore, even the remaining 5% of this level is still close to that maintaining spermatogenesis in some other species [5, 6, 9]. Secondly, the drop of gonadotropin levels may not be as dramatic as it appears from radioimmunoassay measurements of serum LH and FSH. Indeed, it has been shown by several groups, that there is a discrepancy between immunoreactive and bioactive LH during the treatment; the immunoreactivity shows usually of 50–70% drop whereas the bioactivity decreases over 95% [8, 25]. Our recent findings show that the discrepancy between the immuno/bioactive FSH changes is even greater during this treatment. There is a variable decrease in FSH immunoreactivity during LH-RH agonist treatment [16, 20, 25], but no decrease at all was observed in FSH bioactivity during a 6-month treatment period [13]. These two findings together, the residual testicular testosterone content and the normal circulating FSH bioactivity, may explain the inconsistency of spermatogenic suppression during LH-RH therapy.

In conclusion, our direct measurements of effects of long term LH-RH agonist treatment on the human testis tissue have revealed that although testicular androgen production is effectively suppressed, the steroidogenesis per se is not totally blocked. Production of several steroid precursor of androgens continue. Likewise, the capability of the testis tissue to respond to gonadotropin stimulation is maintained. The residual steroidogenic activity of the testis may not compromise the therapeutic effect of the treatment in prostatic cancer. However, in the face of unaffected secretion of bioactive FSH [13], it may explain the incomplete suppression of spermatogenesis by this treatment. Since LH-RH agonists have also prospects for a male contraceptive agent, it will be important to explore whether more efficient pituitary suppression (e.g. that of prolactin and bioactive FSH) will result in more complete blockade of testicular endocrine and spermatogenic functions.

References

[1] Bartsch, W., C. Knabbe, K.-D. Voigt: Regulation and compartmentalization of androgens in rat prostate and muscle. J. Steroid Biochem. **19** (1983) 929 – 937.
[2] Bhasin, S., D. Heber, B. S. Steiner et al.: Hormonal effects of gonadotropin-releasing hormone (GnRH) agonist in the human male. III. Effects of long-term combined treatment with GnRH agonist and androgen. J. Clin. Endocrinol. Metab. **60** (1985) 998 – 1003.
[3] Bhasin, S., R. S. Swerdloff: Mechanisms of gonadotropin-releasing hormone agonist action in the human male. Endocr. Rev. 7 (1986) 106 – 114.
[4] Clayton, R. N., I. T. Huhtaniemi: Absence of gonadotropin-releasing hormone receptors in humand gonadal tissue. Nature **299** (1982) 56 – 59.
[5] Cunningham, G. R., C. Huckins: Persistence of complete spermatogenesis in the presence of low intratesticular concentrations of testosterone. Endocrinology **105** (1979) 177 – 186.
[6] Desjardins, C., L. L. Ewing, D. C. Irby: Response of the rabbit seminiferous epithelium to testosterone administered via polydimethylsiloxane capsules. Endocrinology **93** (1973) 450 – 460.
[7] Doelle, G. C., N. Alexander, R. M. Evans et al.: Combined treatment with LH-RH agonist and testosterone in man: Reversible ologospermia without impotence. J. Androl. **4** (1983) 298 – 302.
[8] Evans, R. M., G. C. Doelle, J. Lindner at al.: A luteinizing hormone-releasing hormone agonist decreases activity and modifies chromatographic behaviour of luteinizing hormone in man. J. Clin. Invest. 73 (1984) 262 – 266.
[9] Ewing, L. L., B. R. Zirkin, R. C. Chochran et al.: Testosterone secretion by rat, rabbit, guinea pig, dog, and hamster testes perfused in vitro: Correlation with Leydig cell mass. Endocrinology **105** (1979) 1135 – 1142.
[10] Hsueh, A. J. W., P. B. C. Jones: Extrapituitary actions of gonadotropin-releasing hormone. Endocr. Rev. **2** (1981) 437 – 461.
[11] Huhtaniemi, I., N. Bolton, P. Leinonen et al.: Testicular luteinizing hormone receptor content and in vitro stimulation of cyclic adenosine 3′,5′-monophosphate and steroid production: A comparison between man and rat. J. Clin. Endocrinol. Metab. **55** (1982) 882 – 889.
[12] Huhtaniemi, I. T., K. J. Catt: Induction and maintenance of gonadotropin and lactogen receptors in hypoprolactinemic rats. Endocrinology **109** (1981) 483 – 490.
[13] Huhtaniemi, I. T., K. D. Dahl, S. Rannikko et al.: Serum bioactive and immunoreactive follicle-stimulating hormone in prostatic cancer patients during GnRH agonist treatment and after orchidectomy. J. Clin. Endocrinol. Metab., 1988, in press.
[14] Huhtaniemi, I., H. Nikula, M. Parvinen et al.: Histological and functional changes of the testis tissue during GnRH agonist treatment of prostatic cancer. Proceedings of the 14th International Cancer Congress, Budapest, 1986 (In press).
[15] Huhtaniemi, I., H. Nikula, S. Rannikko: Treatment of prostatic cancer with a gonadotropin-releasing hormone agonist analog: Acute and long term effects on endocrine functions of testis tissue. J. Clin. Endocrinol. Metab. **61** (1985) 698 – 704.
[16] Huhtaniemi, I., H. Nikula, M. Parvinen et al.: Pituitary-testicular function of prostatic cancer patients during treatment with a GnRH agonist analog: 2. Endocrinology and histology of the testis tissue. J. Androl. **8** (1987) 363 – 373.
[17] Huhtaniemi, I., H. Nikula, S. Rannikko: Pituitary-testicular function of prostatic cancer patients during treatment with a GnRH agonist analog: I. Circulating hormone levels. J. Androl. **8** (1987) 355 – 362.
[18] Huhtaniemi, I. T., J. M. Stewart, K. Channabasavaiah et al.: Effect of treatment with GnRH antagonist, GnRH antiserum and bromocriptine on pituitary-testicular function of adult rats. Mol. Cell Endocrinol. **34** (1984) 127 – 135.
[19] Johnson, S. G.: Testicular biopsy score count – A method for registration of spermatogenesis in human testes: Normal values and results in 335 hypogonadal males. Hormones **1** (1970) 2 – 25.
[20] Labrie, F., A. Dupont, A. Belanger (eds.): LHRH and its analogues. Basic and clinical aspects, pp. 1 – 541. Excerpta Medica, Amsterdam 1985.

[21] Linde, R., G. C. Doelle, N. Alexander et al.: Reversible inhibition of testicular steroidogenesis and spermatogenesis by a potent gonadotropin-releasing hormone agonist in normal men. N. Engl. J. Med. **305** (1981) 663–667.
[22] The Leuprolide Study Group. Leuprolide versus diethylstilbestrol for metastatic prostatic cancer. N. Engl. J. Med. **311** (1984) 1281–1286.
[23] Martikainen, H., I. Huhtaniemi, R. Vihko: Response of peripheral serum sex steroids and some of their precursors to a single injection of hCG in adult men. Clin. Endocr. **13** (1980) 157–166.
[24] Parmer, H., R. H. Phillips, S. L. Lightman et al.: Randomised controlled study of orchiectomy vs long-acting D-Trp-6-LHRH microcapsules in advanced prostate carcinoma. Lancet **II** (1985) 1201–1205.
[25] Warner, B., T. J. Worgul, J. Drago et al.: Effect of very high dose D-leucine^{6}-gonadotropin-releasing hormone proethylamide on the hypothalamic-pituitary testicular axis in patients with prostatic cancer. J. Clin. Invest. **71** (1983) 1842–1853.

Animal models for prostate cancer

U. Otto, B. Wagner, G. Klöppel, H. Baisch, H. Klosterhalfen

Introduction

For the investigation of basic biological patterns of tumors animal models are essential. Knowledge about basic functions and properties of malignant tumors cannot be obtained by clinical studies alone. On the other side in vitro experiments just allow to study single aspects of the tumor without all the various influences of its natural environment. Few culture cell lines were derived from human prostate cancer. In many cases overgrowth by fibroblasts was observed [11, 6]. Therefore many attempts have been made to establish suitable animal models for the investigation of prostatic cancer. Due to different reasons these models are unable to answer most basic questions about the pathophysiology of prostatic tumors [4].

For example two very well known animal models are the Dunning tumor in rats [1] and the Noble rat prostate carcinoma [5], which have been used to evaluate many biochemical modalities in malignant prostate tissue, but they both are not of human origin. Therefore their usefulness is limited. The investigation of human tumors requires viable, growing human tumor tissue containing all different cell types in their natural environment and the possibility to manipulate its environmental conditions. This led to many efforts to establish human tumor cell lines by transplantation into animals.

First attempts were made avoiding host versus graft reactions by implanting the human tumor tissue into immunologically inert sites of the animals such as the eye chamber or the brain of the host animals. Prostate cancer never has been successfully transplanted into these sites [11].

Another way to provide the graft from rejection was the use of millipore chambers. The tumor tissue was fixed in a chamber with pores, which were big enough to allow nutritional supply but no cells of the host animal could enter the chamber causing rejection of the tissue. This model was used successfully for several tumors, but prostate carcinoma did not grow in these chambers [11].

A more promising model was established by implantation of human tumors into the cheekpouch of immunosuppressed hamsters. Immunosuppression was ob-

New Developments in Biosciences 4

tained by irradiation or medical treatment of the animals [11]. No prostate cancer was grown in this model.

Finally Williams and co-workers [18] succeeded in growing malignant prostate tissue after transplantation into immunosuppressed mice. Here also immunosuppression was performed by irradiation of the animals, but their group never obtained a continuous tumor line viable enough to allow subsequent investigations.

Since the immundeficient athymic nude mice are used for animal models, a variety of human tumors has been successfully transplanted into these animals [7, 8]. Anyway the transplantation of many different endocrine tumors caused problems due to letal hormone levels in the mice after transplantation of hormone producing tissue [11]. On the other side hormone dependent tumors are not well accepted by the animals without substitution of their essential hormones [2]. Especially prostate cancer has very low acceptance rates [11]. We therefore aimed to establish prostate cancer lines in nude mice.

Material and methods

Tissue from 12 patients with prostate cancer was transplanted into NMRI nu/nu mice. The tissue was obtained from 12 patients in the clinic of Urology, University of Hamburg. 4 × radical prostatectomy was performed, 1 × transurethral resection. In 5 patients metastatic lymphnodes were exstirpated and in 2 cases we used tissue obtained by pouch needle biopsy. The NMRI nu/nu mice, 3 and 6 – 8 weeks old, were kept in laminar flow chambers at 27 C and 55% humidity. They were fed with Altromin and water ad libitum.

After obtaining the prostate tissue from the patients, one representative part was developed for routine histological determination. The remainder was then minced and incubated in TC 199 culture medium (Behring, FRG). Pieces of 3 × 3 × 3 mm (except for needle biopsy material) were then immediately implanted subcutaneously on both sides of the anterior thoracic wall of the mice under sterile conditions. The tissue obtained by needle biopsy was implanted completely.

Then tumor-growth was measured weekly and tumor doubling-time was determined using the transformed Gompertz-function according to Spang-Thomsen [13]. All samples for the histological determinations, prostate tumors and their transplants, were fixed and stained with hematoxylin-eosin using routine methods. Additionally some samples were stained with fluorescent PSA antibodies. DNA-content and number of proliferating cells were determined by flow-cytometry as described earlier by our group [9]. Androgen receptors were measured according to Wagner [16].

Statistical evaluations were performed using the students T-test and correlations were calculated by chi-square-tests.

Results

In all cases vital tumor tissue was found even 4–6 months after transplantation of the prostate cancer tissue into the nude mice. Only 3 out of 12 tumors were finally accepted by the animals. These 3 tumor lines grew progrediently and after sufficient tumor growth were retransplanted for further passages (tab. 1).

Table 1 Transplantation of human prostate cancer tissue into nude mice

Nr.	Patient	Age	Stage	Surgery	Grade	Nr. of pass.	progred. grouth
1	E.O.	G1	D1	RP	II	1	−
2	H.W.	71	D2	LE	III	1	−
3	S.M.	54	D2	LE	IV	1	−
4	R.M.	64	B	RP	I	3	+
5	S.H.	68	D2	LE	IV	2	−
6	P.K.	67	B	RP	II	23	+
7	E.K.	67	B	RP	I	7	−
8	W.I.	59	D	LE	IV	18	+
9	N.D.	60	D	SB	II	2	−
10	R.O.	76	C	SB	II	3	+
11	G.J.	65	D2	LE	IV	3	+
12	M.F.	87	C	TUR	III	3	+

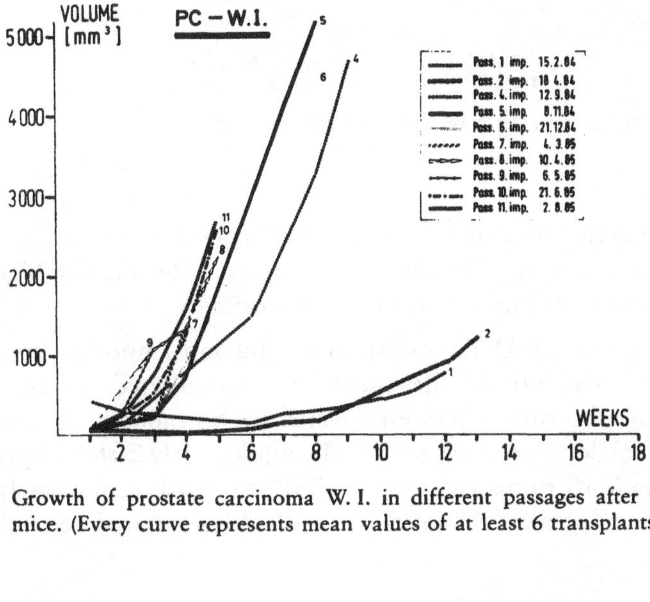

Fig. 1 Growth of prostate carcinoma W. I. in different passages after transplantation into nude mice. (Every curve represents mean values of at least 6 transplants of the same tumor.)

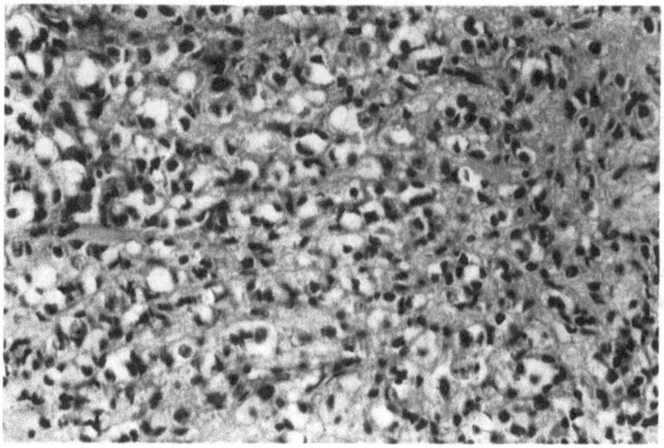

Fig. 2 Lymphnode metastasis of prostate carcinoma.

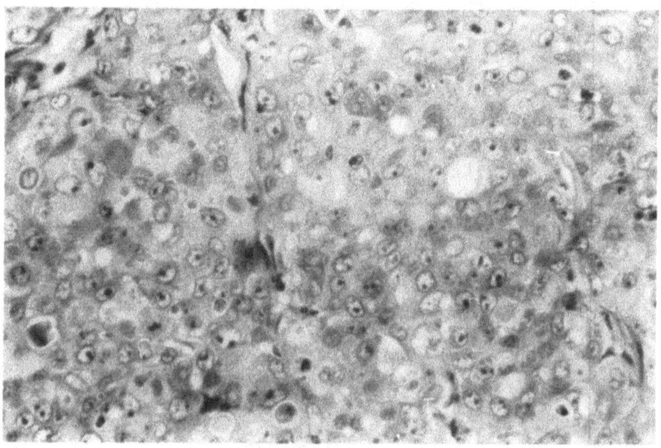

Fig. 3 Same lymphnode metastasis after transplantation into nude mice.

After several passages in the mice all 3 lines expressed growth acceleration, tumor doubling-time decreased (fig. 1). The acceptance seems to be slightly higher in the 3 weeks old mice when compared to the elderly ones.

5alpha-dihydrotestosterone (5a-DHT) substitution did not improve tumor acceptance. Growth and viability of the tissue was not altered by hormonal stimulation. Obviously all 3 tumor lines established are hormone insensitive. No androgen receptors were detected in the tissue. Morphologically 2 of the 3 prostate cancers were solid grade III tumors, 1 was a cribriform grade II tumor. During several passages in the nude mice the grade II tumor differentiated better (grade

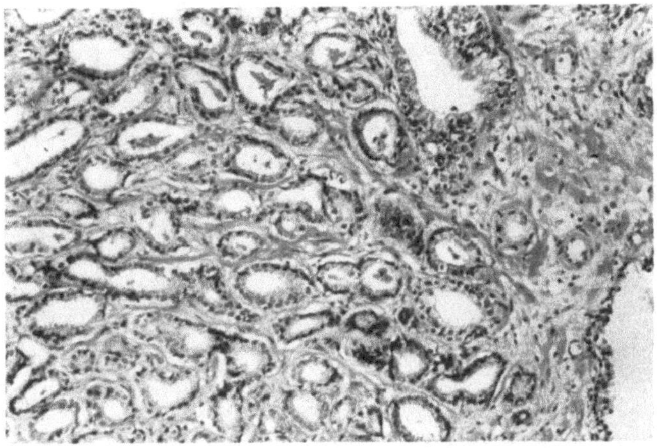

Fig. 4 Prostate carcinoma (grade II) after removal from the patient.

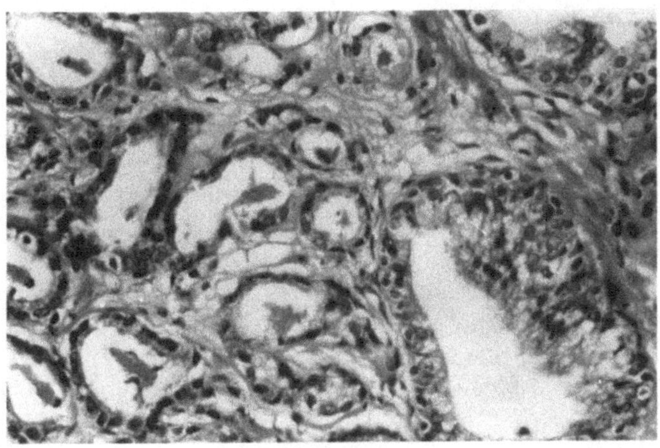

Fig. 5 The same prostate carcinoma (fig. 4) differentiated to grade I after transplantation into nude mice.

I), whereas the other tumors dedifferentiated completely. The histological pettern of the tumors and their transplants are shown in figures 2–5. Significant alterations of the DNA-index during several passages were determined by flow cytometry. An example is shown in figure 6.

No correlation was found between the tumor grade and acceptance-rate, tumor doubling time or number of possible passages after retransplantation. The number of proliferating cells in the tumors correlated well with the clinical tumor stage in the patient and the number of possible passages in the mice.

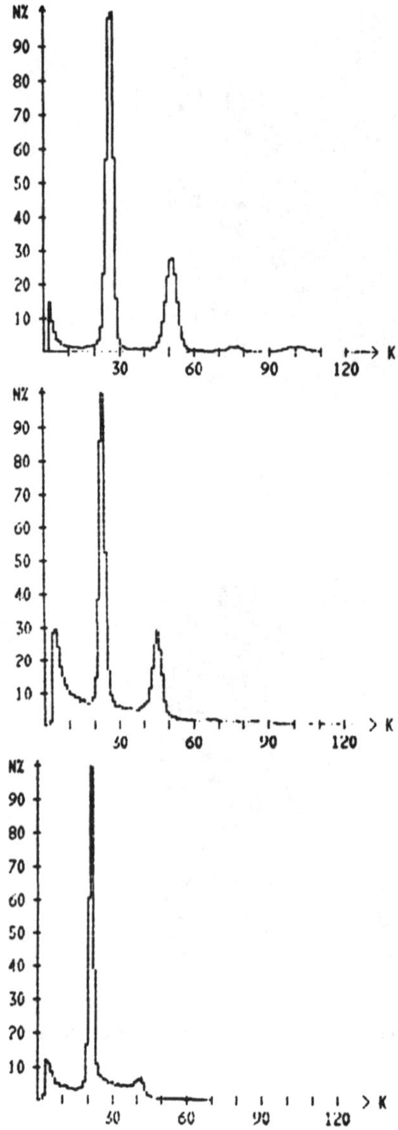

Fig. 6 Results of flow-cytometry in prostate cancer tissue after transplantation into nude mice.

Discussion

Several in vitro and in vivo models have been established to study prostate cancer. Cell culturing was performed by many authors, but the tumor cells were either overgrown by fibroblasts or lost their specific potencies due to dedifferentiation under cell culture conditions. Reid and co-workers [12] explain this effect by a lack of intercellular substances, growth factors, when the cells grow in clones without their natural environment.

This problem can be avoided by studying prostate tumors in vivo. This means, that animal models are essential. The Dunning tumor and the Noble rat prostate carcinoma are well described prostate tumors in animals, but they are not of human origin [1, 5]. All results from studies with these models cannot be transferred to the human situation uncritically. Therefore trials were performed to study human prostatic cancer under in vivo conditions. Since transplantation of human prostate tumors into irradiated animals was not successful, the nude mouse, an ideal acceptor of xenografts, was chosen as a new model [10, 2]. We were able to establish 3 new prostate cancer tumors lines in the NMRI nu/nu mouse. These hormone insensitive tumors represent the therapy resistent type of prostate cancer.

Up to the data of the literature two anaplastic prostate carcinoma cell lines have already been established in nude mice by Mickey and co-workers [3], but these cell lines were grown in vitro for 13 and 60 passages before injection into the mice. Reid and co-workers [12] succeded in establishing 1 hormone sensitive prostatic tumor line (R 198) after transplantation of more than 100 prostatic specimens into nude mice. Schroeder and Steenbrugge [15] established several human prostatic cell lines in the nude mouse. The PC 82, which also is hormone dependent, is used for investigations of the hormone dependent type of prostate cancer. Two other prostate cancer lines have been recently established in nude mice by Schrott and co-workers [17].

Acceptance rates for prostate cancer tissue in nude mice are very low. The reason for this low acceptance rate of prostatic tumors after transplantation into nude mice remains unclear. Of curse hormone substitution for hormone dependent tumors is necessary, but the tumor acceptance in the mice is low for both, hormone sensitive and hormone insensitive tumors. In conclusion there must be other factors but hormones influencing tumor growth after transplantation. 4 more possible reasons for this phenomenon are discussed.

Since in our experiments the acceptance of the tumors seems to be slightly better in very young mice (3 weeks old), the low acceptance rates might be due to the development of natural killer cells in the elderly ones. A certain role of natural killer cells has already been presumed by Reid [12]. This is a possible explanation for the fact, that metastatic growth of the tumors is not frequently observed in the mice. On the other side a lack of essential human growth factors in the mice cannot be excluded [11]. Regarding the fact that tumor acceptance in the mice is extremely variable for different tumor tissues, it may be concluded, that nude mice can suppress growth of tumors with certain antigenic properties. Last not least Stamey and other investigators contribute the low acceptance rate to the low proliferative tendency of prostatic tissue when compared to other malignant tumors [14].

Our own results do not support this hypothesis. The findings from flow cytometry show that the percentage of cells in the different cell cycle phases is variable in prostate tumors. Different cell clones in the heterogenous prostate cancer are able to change dominance and therefore growth acceleration occurs after several passages (fig. 6). Additionally tumor growth is influenced by differences in vascularisation and the velocity of cell death.

The clinical treatment of advanced prostate cancer by androgen deprivation is limited by the well known escape phenomenon. In many cases initial remission of the tumor is followed by sudden occurence of progressive disease due to the loss of hormone sensitivity in the tumors. Therefore investigation of the tumor insensitive and up to date incurable type of prostate cancer is very important and might help us to find new therapeutic regimens for the hormone independent prostate cancer.

The present animal model is useful to clarify nature and properties of polyclonal tumors. Either environmental conditions lead to adaptation of the tumors by selection of clones or by alterations in the genome. Growth acceleration of the tumors after several passages as well as our results in flow-cytometry and histopathology prove the polyclonality of the 3 tumor lines.

The effects of different therapy regimes on different parts of polyclonal prostate cancer tissue can be studied to explain the escape phenomenon and lead to better therapy.

References

[1] Dunning, W. F.: Prostate cancer in the rat. Nat. Cancer Inst., Monogr. **12** (1963) 351.

[2] Kleine, W.: Die thzmusaplastische nu/nu Maus als in-vivo-Testmodell. In: G. A. Nagel, R. Sauer, H. W. Schreiber (eds.): Aktuelle Onkologie 17. W. Zuckschwerdt Verlag, München, Bern, Wien 1985.

[3] Mickey, D. D., K. R. Stone, H. Wunderli et al.: Heterotransplantation of a human prostatic adenocarcinoma cell line in nude mice. Cancer Research **37** (1977) 4049–4057.

[4] Murphy, G. P.: Progress in clinical and biological research: models for prostate cancer. Alan Liss, New York 1980.

[5] Noble, R. L.: The development of prostatic adenocarcinoma in the Nb rat following prolonged sex hormone administration. Cancer res. **37** (1977) 1929–1933.

[6] Okada, K., F. H. Schröder: Human prostatic carcinoma in cell culture: preliminary report on the development and characterization of epithelial cell lines (EB-33). Urol. Res. **2** (1974) 111.

[7] Otto, U., G. Klöppel, H. Baisch: Transplantation of human renal cell carcinoma into NMRI nu/nu mice. I. The reliability of an experimental tumor model. J. Urol. **131** (1984) 134.

[8] Otto, U., H. Baisch, G. Klöppel: Malignancy Index based on flow cytometry and histology for renal cell carcinomas and its correlation to prognosis. J. Urol. **135**, No. 247 (1986) 165 A.

[9] Otto, U., H. Baisch, H. Huland et al.: Tumor cell DNA content and prognosis in human renal cell carcinoma. J. Urol. **132** (1984) 237.
[10] Povlson, C. O., J. Rygaard: Heterotransplantation of human adenocarcinoma of the colon and rectum to the mouse mutant nude. A study of nine consecutive transplantations. Acta path. microbiol. scand. Sect. A, **79** (1971) 159.
[11] Reid, M.: Transplantation of heterologous endocrine tumor cells in nude mice, pp. 313–352. Academic Press, New York, San Francisco, London 1978.
[12] Reid, M., J. Holland, C. Jones et al.: Some of the variables affecting the success of transplantation of human tumors into the athymic nude mouse. In: D. P. Houches, A. A. Ovejera (eds.): Proceedings of the symposium on the use of athymic (nude) mice in cancer research, pp. 107. G. Fischer Verlag, New York, Stuttgart 1978.
[13] Spang-Thomsen, M., A. Nielsen, J. Visfeld: Growth curves of three human malignant tumors transplanted to nude mice. Exp. Cell Biol. **48** (1980) 138.
[14] Stamey, T. A.: Cancer of the prostate: Monography in Urology. Vol. **4**, No. 3 (1983) 65.
[15] Steenbrugge, G. J., M. Groen, J. C. Romijn et al.: Biological effects of hormonal treatment regimes on a transplantable human prostatic tumor line (PC-82). J. Urol. **131** (1984) 812–817.
[16] Wagner, R. K.: Characterization and assay of steroid hormone receptors and steroid-binding serum proteins by agargel-electrophoresis at low temperature. Hoppe-Seyler's 2. Physiol. Chem. **353** (1972) 1235.
[17] Walther, M.: Entwicklung und vergleichende experimentelle Hormontherapie der menschlichen Prostata-Karzinom-Tumorlinie PC EW auf der Nacktmaus. Dissertation der Friedrich-Alexander-Universität Erlangen-Nürnberg.
[18] Williams, G., R. Ghanadian, J. E. Castro: The growth and viability of human prostatic tissue maintained in immunosuppressed mice. Clinical Oncology **4** (1978) 347–351.

The significance of the nude mice model for studies on human prostatic carcinoma

G. J. van Steenbrugge, F. H. de Jong, M. P. W. Gallee, F. H. Schröder

Introduction

Since the discovery of Huggins and Hodges that prostatic cancer could be made to regress by either orchiectomy or by the administration of exogenous estrogens, the treatment of advanced prostatic cancer has depended upon the suppression of circulating levels of androgens [16]. The standard forms of endocrine management do not completely eliminate plasma androgens. Some investigators suggest that a more complete form of androgen withdrawal, in which the low levels of non-testicular androgens are counteracted, might be more effective than castration alone [9]. The validity of this suggestion strongly depends on the answer to the question what minimal amount of androgen is necessary to support tumor growth. Using the hormone-dependent subline of the Dunning R3327 prostatic tumor in the rat the optimal concentration of circulating testosterone (T) which should be reached in the treatment of prostatic cancer has been determined [1, 14]. Information about the effects of varying concentrations of circulating T and the growth of human prostatic cancer tissue can only be obtained by the use of tumor models of human origin. Among the limited number of prostatic tumor lines established in nude mice, the PC-82 [6], PC-EW [7], Honda [8] and TEN/12 tumors [5] were shown to be androgen-dependent. The PC-82 tumor model, which was established in our own institution [6] shares several properties with clinical prostatic carcinoma and was shown to be an appropriate model to study the effects of hormonal treatment on human prostatic cancer tissue [11]. We have succeeded in maintaining constant physiological levels of plasma T in nude mice [10, 12] as well as in administering pharmacological doses of estradiol to PC-82 tumor-bearing mice [13] by using Silastic implants filled with testosterone or estradiol respectively. However, the release rate of steroids from these implants appeared to be too high to obtain low (near-castrate) levels of circulating androgen. Therefore, in the present study with the PC-82 tumor various low levels of plasma T were maintained by implantation of Silastic capsules containing different proportions of T mixed with cholesterol.

New Developments in Biosciences 4

Recently, a monoclonal antibody Ki-67 was described [3] which identifies a proliferation associated nuclear antigen. As marker this antigen was shown to be suitable to detect early responses of the PC-82 tumor to hormonal manipulation [2]. This contribution describes the use of this proliferation marker to monitor time-dependent effects of hormonal manipulation on the PC-82 tumor. Furthermore, we tried to correlate tissue androgen levels with the percentage of Ki-67 positive cells in tissue specimens of the same tumor.

Materials and methods

PC-82 tumor

The transplantable human prostate carcinoma, PC-82, was maintained in Balb/c nude mice obtained from our breeding colony. Details about the technique of transplantation and of the way tumor growth was monitored have been described previously [11]. The present experiments were carried out with tumors of the 30–35th transplant generation.

Hormonal manipulation

Castration was carried out via the scrotal route under total anesthesia with tribromoethanol (Aldrich, Beerse, Belgium). Testosterone (Steraloids, Pawling, NY) was administered by using subcutaneously implanted Silastic capsules, releasing the steroid at a constant rate, as described before [10]. To obtain low levels of circulating T in the nude mice Silastic implants were prepared containing different proportions of T mixed with cholesterol. For these "hormonal-titration" experiments the implants were made of Silastic tubing (Talas, Zwolle, Netherlands) of 1.5 mm inner and 2.1 mm outer diameter. The implants had a length of 1.0 cm of which 0.6 cm tubing was effectively filled with steroid. Installation of the implants was carried out under light ether anesthesia.

Immunocytochemistry

The immunocytochemical procedure with the murine Ki-67 monoclonal antibody (Dakopatts, Denmark) was performed either on cryostat sections or on fine-needle aspiration material. Fine-needle aspiration biopsies were taken from tumor-bearing mice without anesthesia by using a 20 ml disposable syringe in a special holder (Cameco, 20 ml, Precision Dynamics, Burbank, CA). Smears, which have been made directly after taking the aspirate, were subsequently air-dried (1 h), fixed in acetone for 10 min and stored at $-20°$ C. The further procedure was similar to that described by Gallee et al. [2].

Miscellaneous

At the end of the hormonal-titration experiments the remaining tumor-bearing mice were exsanguinated from the orbital sinus under ether anesthesia. Plasma was obtained by centrifugation at 9000 g for 3 min and stored at −20° C until analysis. The concentration of androgens in PC-82 tumor tissue was estimated as previously described [12]. The concentration of T in the plasma of the mice was estimated by radioimmunoassay by using the method and antiserum described by Verjans et al. [15]. The significance of differences between values of different groups was calculated using two-tailed Student's T-tests.

Results

Hormone-dependence

The absence of PC-82 tumor growth in intact female and in castrated male nude mice indicates the absolute requirement of androgens for the growth of this

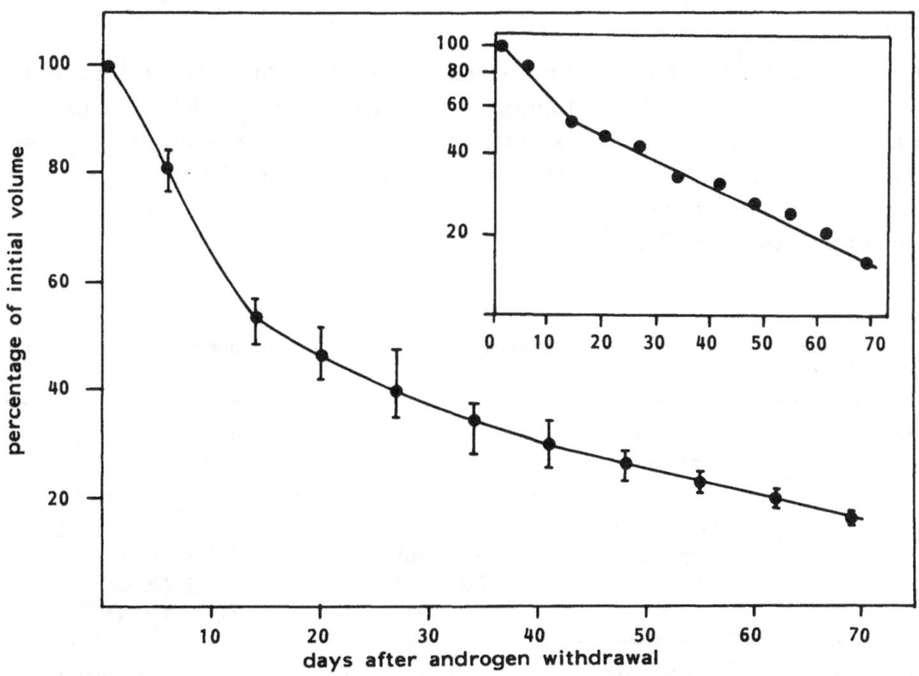

Fig. 1 The effect of castration and/or removal of T-implant on the PC-82 prostatic tumor grown in intact and in T-implanted male nude mice.
Values are expressed as mean ± S. E. M. (n = 8). Inset shows the semilogarithmic plot of the data.

tumor. The castration-induced regression of the tumor resulted in a 80% reduction of the tumor volume at 70 days after androgen withdrawal (fig. 1). The plot of the log of tumor volume versus days after castration (fig. 1; inset) demonstrates a biphasic curve. An initial period of 14 days with a relatively rapid rate of regression is followed by a more gradual but also exponential rate of tumor reduction (times of half-life 15 and 32 days respectively).

Plasma levels of testosterone

To improve the take and growth of the PC-82 tumor and to facilitate hormonal manipulation in tumor-bearing mice, a standard T implant (length: 1.0 cm) was used. Implantation of male and female mice with this type of T capsule resulted in an average plasma T concentration of 25 nmol/l. In contrast to the small variation of plasma T levels in T-implanted male mice, intact male mice showed a wide range of circulating T-levels varying from less than 1.0 nmol/l to levels exceeding 90 nmol/l.

Growth-stimulating effect of different levels of circulating androgen

T-implants containing different proportions of T mixed with cholesterol, resulting in plasma T levels of 0.2 – 19.4 nmol/l, were applied to PC-82 transplanted, castrated male nude mice. The take rate (i. e. the percentage of tumors reaching the volume of 100 mm^3) in mice supported with 25% T-implants was found to be similar to that of tumors receiving 100% T-implants (tab. 1). Tumor tissue transplanted in the 10% T-group had a considerably lower take (40%) and finally

Table 1 Growth of PC-82 tumor tissue transplanted in castrated male mice supplemented with different doses of testosterone (T)*

Proportion of T in the implant (%)	Final T-level (nmol/l)	Tumor take (%)	Tv (mm3)
0	0.7 ± 0.4 (4)	0 (0/8)	–
10	1.8 ± 0.3 (3)	40 (4/10)	127 ± 53 (4)[a]
25	4.0 ± 0.7 (4)	70 (10/14)	239 ± 126 (9)[b]
100	7.0 (2)	79 (11/14)	742 ± 436 (11)

* Values represent means ± S.D. (number of observations). Tumor take (the point tumors had reached the volume of 100 mm^3 and tumor volume (Tv) of the tumors were determined at 90 days after transplantation.

a) Significantly different from 100% T-group ($P < 0.01$)

b) Significantly different from 100% T-group ($P < 0.02$)

in the control mice receiving implants with 100% cholesterol no tumor growth was observed. The mean tumor volume reached at 90 days after transplantation of tumors in the 10% and 25% T-implanted mice was significantly smaller in comparison with tumors in the 100% T-supported animals. The difference between the tumor volume in the 10% and 25% implanted mice was not statistically significant (table 1).

Effect of hormonal manipulation on tissue proliferation

The short-term effects of hormonal manipulation on PC-82 tumor tissue in an individual tumor-bearing mouse could be monitored by application of the Ki-67 antibody to cytological specimens of sequentially performed fine-needle biopsies. The percentage of Ki-67 positive cells in a tumor sample, i. e. the total fraction of "cycling" cells expressing the proliferation-associated antigen, decreased from around 14 per cent at the start of the experiment to 0 per cent at 9 days after androgen withdrawal (table 2). Supplementation of androgen by T-implantation in this animal resulted in an increase of the proliferative fraction and the control value had been reached within 12 days after androgen resubstitution.

Table 2 The effect of hormonal manipulation on the expression of a proliferation associated antigen in cytological specimens obtained by sequential aspiration of one individual PC-82 tumor grown in an intact male mouse*

sample	total number of nuclei counted	Ki-67 positive nuclei (%)
T0	511	69 (13.5)
T2−	500	11 (2.2)
T9−	500	0 (0)
T9−/2+	535	15 (2.8)
T9−/12+	510	67 (13.1)

* The animal was hormonally manipulated by castration and testosterone (T)-substitution respectively.
T0: control tumor; (−): duration of T-withdrawal in days; (+): duration of T-resubstitution in days.

Tissue sections derived from the same tumors in which the concentration of dihydrotestosterone (DHT) had been determined (results described previously; cf. ref. 12) were stained with the Ki-67 antibody. Figure 2 illustrates that the relationship between the concentration of DHT and the percentage of Ki-67 positive cells had the feature of an "S-shaped" curve. Clearly two groups of

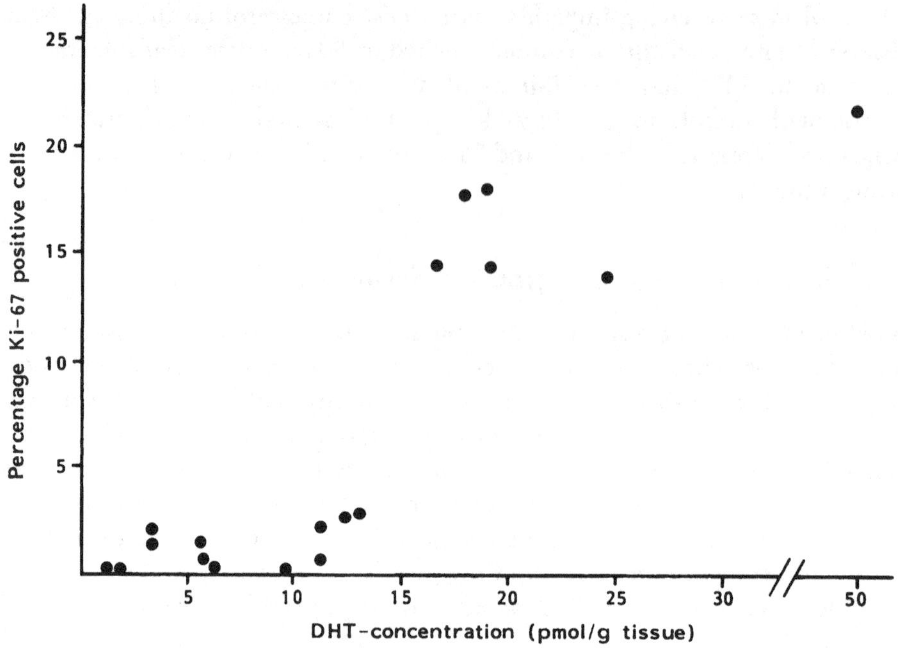

Fig. 2 The relationship between the tumor cell proliferative fraction, determined by the Ki-67 antibody method, and the concentration of DHT in PC-82 tissue grown in T-implanted hormonally manipulated female mice.

tissues can be distinguished. Below the concentration of 15 pmol/g tissue the fraction of Ki-67 positive cells did not exceed 5 per cent, whereas above this concentration at least 14 per cent of the cells expressed the proliferation antigen.

Discussion

Although some new models for human prostate cancer have been established during the last few years, the total number of models demonstrating a hormone-dependent pattern of growth is still limited [5, 7, 8]. The human prostatic carcinoma PC-82 has been maintained in nude mice for 10 years now and passed through 35 transplant generations. The pattern of regression of the PC-82 tumor after androgen withdrawal follows a biphasic course (fig. 1). In none of the long-term castration experiments, with postcastration periods of over 100 days, spontaneous regrowth of the PC-82 tumor was observed. Therefore, it was concluded that this tumor consists of a rather homogeneous population of hormone-responsive cells.

By the use of Silastic implants filled with different proportions of T mixed with cholesterol "hormonal-titration" experiments in the PC-82 tumor were performed. It was found that a plasma T level between 1 and 2 nmol/l (obtained by 10% T-implants) is the threshold below which growth of the PC-82 tumor is no longer stimulated (tab. 1). These data are supported by the observation that PC-82 tumor did not grow in intact female and in castrated male mice in which plasma T did not exceed the level of 1.1 nmol/l. The present results with the PC-82 human prostate model agree fairly well with recent observations with the Dunning R3327 prostate tumor in the rat. By using hormone-dependent sublines of this model it was shown that plasma T levels must be kept below 1.7 nmol/l but do not have to be suppressed to levels lower than 1 nmol/l in order to obtain a maximal suppressive effect on the growth of the tumor [1]. These observations as well as the present findings of the PC-82 tumor support the conclusion that relatively low androgen levels remaining after castration-induced androgen deprivation do not have biological significance with regard to prostatic (tumor) growth. Thus, from the studies of experimental tumors no evidence has been obtained sofar that the approach of total androgen blockade, i. e. surgical or chemical castration combined with anti-androgen treatment to counteract the effects of adrenal androgens [cf. ref. 9] is preferable to the concept of partial androgen withdrawal which can be achieved by castration alone.

The outcome of preliminary experiments dealing with application of the Ki-67 antibody to aspiration biopsy material from PC-82 tumors (tab. 2) as well as the results which have previously been reported [2], indicate that the Ki-67 marker provides a reliable method to estimate the proliferative fraction of hormone-responsive prostate cancer. Gerdes et al. [4] showed that the antigen, which is recognized by the Ki-67 antibody, is expressed in G1, S, G2, and M-phase of all continuously cycling cells but is absent in G0 cells. Therefore, the fraction of Ki-67 positive cells (found to be maximally 30 per cent) in PC-82 tumor tissues are to be considered as the fraction of cycling cells of this tumor.

The continuing experiments with low-dose androgen substitution in the PC-82 and other hormone-dependent human tumor models in nude mice will include concomitant measurements of endogenous androgen levels and the proliferative fraction of the tissues. Such studies will yield valuable information on the relationship between androgens and growth of prostatic cancer tissue.

Acknowledgements

The authors wish to acknowledge Mrs. Marja Groen and Mrs. Anjo van Kreuningen for their capable assistance in attending to many aspects of the nude mice work. We thank Mrs. Winny Lotze-Ruizendaal for excellent secretarial assistance.

This study was supported partly by the Stichting Urologisch Wetenschappelijk Onderzoek (SUWO) and by the Netherlands Cancer Foundation (KWF) through grant IKR 87.8.

References

[1] Ellis, W. J., J. T. Isaacs: Effectiveness of complete versus partial androgen withdrawal therapy for treatment of prostatic cancer as studied in the Dunning R3327 system of rat prostatic adenocarcinomas. Cancer res. **45** (1985) 6041 – 6050.

[2] Gallee, M. P. W., G. J. van Steenbrugge, F. J. W. ten Kate et al.: Determination of proliferative fraction of a transplantable hormone-dependent human prostatic carcinoma (PC-82) by the monoclonal antibody Ki-67; potential application for hormone therapy monitoring. J. Natl. Cancer Inst. **79** (1987) 1333 – 1340.

[3] Gerdes, J., U. Schwab, H. Lemke et al.: Production of a mouse monoclonal antibody reactive with a human nuclear antigen associated with cell proliferation. Int. J. Can. **31** (1983) 13 – 20.

[4] Gerdes, J., H. Lemke, H. Baisch et al.: Cell cycle analysis of a cell proliferation-associated human nuclear antigen defined by the monoclonal antibody Ki-67. J. Immunol. **133** (1984) 1710 – 1715.

[5] Harper, M. E., P. E. C. Sibley, A. Rowlands et al.: Hormonal modulation of the growth of a new transplantable prostatic cell line in athymic nude mice. Urol. Res. **14**(1986) 156 (abstr.).

[6] Hoehn, W., F. H. Schroeder, J. F. Riemann et al.: Human prostatic adenocarcinoma: some characteristics of a serially transplantable line in nude mice (PC-82). The Prostate **1** (1980) 95 – 104.

[7] Hoehn, W., M. Wagner, J. F. Riemann et al.: Prostatic adenocarcinoma. PC EW, a new human tumor line transplantable in nude mice. The Prostate **5** (1984) 445 – 452.

[8] Ito, Y. Z., S. Mashimo, Y. Nakazato et al.: Hormone dependency of a serially transplantable human prostatic cancer (Honda) in nude mice. Cancer Res. **45** (1985) 5058 – 5063.

[9] Labrie, F., A. Dupont, A. Belanger et al.: New approach in the treatment of prostate cancer: complete instead of partial withdrawal of androgens. The Prostate **4** (1983) 579 – 594.

[10] Steenbrugge, G. J. van, M. Groen, F. H. de Jong et al.: The use of steroid-containing Silastic implants in male nude mice: plasma hormone levels and the effect of implantation on the weights of the ventral prostate and seminal vesicles. The Prostate **5** (1984) 639 – 647.

[11] Steenbrugge, G. J. van, M. Groen, J. C. Romijn et al.: Biological effects of hormonal treatment regimens on a transplantable human prostatic tumor line (PC-82). J. Urol. **131** (1984) 812 – 817.

[12] Steenbrugge, G. J. van, J. J. W. van Dongen, P. J. Reuvers et al.: Transplantable human prostatic carcinoma (PC-82) in athymic nude mice: I. Hormone-dependence and the concentration of androgens in plasma and tumor tissue. The Prostate **11** (1987) 195 – 210.

[13] Steenbrugge, G. J. van, M. Groen, F. H. de Jong et al.: Human prostatic carcinoma (PC-82) in athymic nude mice: III. Effects of estrogens on the growth of tumor tissue. The Prostate (1988), in press.

[14] Trachtenberg, J.: Optimal testosterone concentration for the treatment of prostatic cancer. J. Urol. **133** (1985) 888 – 890.

[15] Verjans, H. L., B. A. Cooke, F. H. de Jong et al.: Evaluation of a radioimmunoassay for testosterone estimation. J. Steroid. Biochem. **4** (1973) 665 – 676.

[16] Walsh, P. C.: Physiologic basis for hormonal therapy in carcinoma of the prostate. Urol. Clin. North. Am. **2** (1975) 125 – 140.

II Etiology and experimental basis of therapy

Etiology and natural history of early prostatic cancer

F. H. Schröder

Introduction

Clinical and epidemiological evidence clearly shows that several steps are involved in the etiology of clinically relevant prostatic carcinoma.

Focal carcinoma is found in autopsy series and surgically resected tissue from BPH with a prevalence which is roughly 500 times higher than the incidence of clinical carcinoma. Focal carcinoma and maybe also the even more frequent dysplasia must be considered precursors of clinical carcinoma. On the other hand most of these tumors never reach the clinical stage. The fact that in some countries (Japan, Singapore) the incidence of the true focal lesions is identical to that in Western countries, whereas the incidence of extensive tumors is much lower, seems to indicate that environmental promoting factors play a role. Epidemiological studies point into the direction of sexual behaviour, diet and the use of vitamins as possibly having an impact.

For the pathogenesis of hormone independent prostatic carcinoma at least three mutational steps seem to be required: normal cell → focal carcinoma → hormone dependent carcinoma → hormone independent carcinoma. There is little indication that endocrine factors play a role in these events, although prostatic carcinoma rarely or never develops in early castrated males.

The natural history of untreated prostatic carcinoma as a consequence of what has been said is at least in its early phase much determined by host factors. It is characterized by the fact that stage progression or persistence occurs in all possible ways. The natural development of tumor extension is paralleled by a change of tumor grade and possibly also of ploidy. Natural history is accompanied by considerable variations in risk which are difficult to predict in the individual.

Clinical prostatic carcinoma originates from focal lesions, focal carcinoma and its precursor dysplasia, which can be microscopically identified within the otherwise normal prostatic tissue. The prevalence of such lesions increases with age and varies between 0 and 80%. The age dependence of focal carcinoma is paralleled by clinical carcinoma, clinical carcinoma, however, becomes relatively

New Developments in Biosciences 4

more frequent above the age of 70 than focal carcinoma. Still, the prevalence of focal lesions independent of age groups is in the range of 500 to 1000 times higher than the mortality of prostatic carcinoma. This strongly suggests, that independent of the time available, not all focal carcinomas developed into clinically detectable lesions. The very large difference in the frequency with which focal lesions and clinical carcinomas occur also suggest that different etiological factors must be responsible for the origination of these two different entities of the same disease. Obviously, it would not make sense to treat all patients who might be identified with focal prostatic carcinoma in an aggressive fashion. This would result in overtreatment in a very large patient population. It is mandatory, however, to identify those patients in time that do show a tendency toward progression to the clinically relevant, especially to metastatic disease.

For the understanding of this contribution it is essential to know the meaning of some technical terms which will be used. Prostatic carcinoma which is found at autopsy is usually called latent carcinoma. If the tumor was extensive and had lead to metastatic disease which was not recognised during the life time of the diseased, the tumor is called occult prostatic carcinoma. Latent carcinoma may be called focal it its volume is very small. A generally accepted definition for what should be called focal carcinoma is urgently needed. Probably the definition offered by Cantrell et al. [5] has been a subject to consensus by most clinicians: tumors that occupy less than 5% of the entire slide surface are called focal (A1), larger tumors are microscopically extensive tumors that are classified A2 if they cannot be palpated on rectal examination. Prostatic carcinoma that is found at the time of histological examination of prostatic specimens removed for the treatment of prostatic hyperplasia (BPH) is called incidental carcinoma if rectal examination was not suspicious. Incidental carcinoma in the frequently used American classification is subdivided into stage A1 and A2 which coincides with the stages T0pT1 and T0pT2 – 3 in the TNM-classification. A1 tumors are usually well differentiated, A2 tumors are often moderately or poorly differentiated.

The prevalence of incidental carcinoma in routine sections of BPH specimens averages 8 to 12% and depends on the age distribution of the patients and on the way the tissue is sectioned and reviewed.

As for other cancers the etiology of prostatic carcinoma is not known. From what has been said above it can however be concluded that several mutational steps are necessary for the development that leads from the normal prostatic cell to hormone unresponsive metastatizing disease. At least three such alterations are necessary that lead to the three different entities with a clearly different genetic background: focal carcinoma, hormone dependent carcinoma and hormone independent carcinoma of the prostate. These steps are accompanied by a morphological development of any given tumor in the direction from well to poorly differentiated. Kastendiek [8] and McNeal [9] have described premalignant lesions that they consider precursors of focal carcinoma. McNeal identifies two types of lesions, the first one consists of intraductal hyperplasia with progressive atypicality, the second one originates from repeated budding and brauching of new acini without nuclear atypicality. These precursor lesions which again seem to be much more frequent than focal carcinoma may represent again a separate entity with a different genetic background.

Epidemiological aspects

Geographical variations in the incidence of clinical prostatic carcinoma have given much insight into the etiology of clinical prostatic cancer. Originally it was thought, that for instance the very low incidence of prostate cancer in Japan might be due to a racial disposition. It was however shown by Akazaki et al. [1] that the incidence of clinical prostatic carcinoma rises in Japanese immigrants to Hawai and to the American mainland. There is general agreement, that the promotion of prostatic cancer to the clinical stage has something to do with life-style and environment. This conclusion is further confirmed by the finding that in autopsy series from various countries with a high or low incidence of clinical carcinoma the prevalence of focal carcinoma is not different. Among several other authors this was clearly shown by Breslow and his co-workers [3]. In the same autopsy studies usually a difference between the prevalence of locally extensive latent carcinoma is found between geographical areas that coincides with the finding of a low or high clinical incidence of prostatic cancer in those countries. By epidemiological studies a number of leads have been identified that are related to a higher or lower incidence of prostatic carcinoma. These are: diet, fat consumption, vitamine A, exposure to heavy metals, sexual habits, smoking and possibly endocrine factors. The initial endocrine dependence of most clinical prostatic carcinomas suggests strongly that the endocrine environment may play some role in the pathogenesis of clinical prostatic carcinoma. This suspicion is further supported by a positive correlation with evidence of higher sexual activity and prostatic cancer incidence. Also, in autopsy studies, a lower incidence of prostatic carcinoma has been demonstrated in patients suffering from cirrhosis of the liver with elevated plasma estrogen levels. However, careful studies including the Dutch/Japanese case controle study of prostatic carcinoma have failed to show that free and bound age corrected plasma testosterone and dihydrotestosterone levels are any different for patients with carcinoma of the prostate and several age matched control groups. There was also no difference between Dutch and Japanese males with prostatic carcinoma. Without any doubt, one major genetic chance is necessary to transfer hormone sensitive prostatic carcinoma to the hormone insensitive state. Whether this step is governed by endocrine changes is still not known.

The natural history of incidental prostatic carcinoma

The prevalence of incidental prostatic carcinoma is lower than the prevalence of latent carcinoma found in autopsy series. Still, the prevalence of incidental prostatic carcinoma (8 – 12%) is still more than 500 times higher than the incidence of clinically relevant prostatic carcinoma. This creates for the clinician, who identifies these tumors in daily practice a difficult problem in deciding which one requires treatment and which one not. Prevalence and incidence figures cannot be expected to coincide. The prevalence of a certain disease indicates a cross section through time and samples pathological findings at a given moment that may have originated during a long period of time. Incidence indicates the proportion of individuals suffering or dying from a given disease during a time period, usually one year. Still, on this background, the progression rates reported for stage A1 incidental carcinoma in the literature are surprisingly high. Data relating to stage A1 and A2 cancer are summarized in table 1. Epstein and co-workers [7] followed 50 patients with focal incidental carcinoma (stage A1) for more than 8 years. Progression was seen in 16%. Blute and co-workers [2] found progression after an average of 10 years in 4 of 15 men with untreated A1 lesions (26%). In contrast, in the series of Cantrell [5] 32% of 122 patients progressed with an average of 4 years of follow-up when a stage A2 was diagnosed as being a tumor that occupies more than 5% of the total slide surface. At the same time only 2% of those patients whose tumor occupied less than 5% of the total slide surface progressed within 4 years.

Table 1 Natural history of incidental carcinoma – A1 and A2

- Epstein et al. (1987): of 50 patients with focal, incidental carcinoma (A1) followed > 8 years 8 (16%) showed progression
- Blute et al. (1987): among 15 men with A1 lesions 4 (26%) progressed after $\bar{x}$ 10 years of follow-up
- Cantrell et al. (1981): 32% of 122 patients progressed within an average of 4 years of follow-up (stage A2)

Clearly, stage A1 and A2 incidental prostatic carcinoma have a different prognosis. During identical time intervals progression rates for the A2 lesion may be expected to be 10 times or more higher than progression rates for true focal disease. Unfortunately no parameters are available to identify those patients in the large group of those having a A1 disease, who will progress. This puts the clinican in a dilemma. A possible answer might be to treat those patients with a A1 lesion that are very young aggressively if a low morbidity treatment modality is available.

Natural history of locally confined clinical carcinoma (category T1 – 2, stage B)

Again the information in the literature on this disease is scarse. In the study of the Veterans Administration Cooperative Urological Research Group (VACURG) reported by Byar [4] 7 of 20 patients with palpable prostatic nodules, who were followed for an average of 7.7 years showed progression under placebo medication (35%).

Whitmore [10] demonstrated progression to stages C and D in 33% and 20% in 45 selected untreated patients with clinical stage B tumors. The average follow-up was 9.7 years. The data are summarized in table 2. Clearly, the progression rates for palpable nodules which are confined to the prostate (stage B, category T1 – 2) are in the range of 35% at 7 years. The risk is higher if compared to the risk of the A1 lesion. The risk of the A2 lesion may be similar to that of stage B disease. As is evident from treatment results, smaller and larger stage B lesions (stage B1 versus B2) must be expected to show higher progression rates.

Table 2 Natural history of locally confined clinical carcinoma (category T1 – 2, Stage B)

- Byar and VACURG (1981): 7 of 20 patients followed for $\bar{x}$ = 7.7 years showed progression (35%) under placebo medication
- Whitmore (1984): in 45 untreated patients with clinical stage B tumors progression to stages C and D occurred in 33 and 20% within $\bar{x}$ = 7.9 years

In considering the natural history of prostatic carcinoma, age plays a very important role, not only because the incidence of this disease is closely related to increasing age, but also because in this age group typically many other diseases threaten the life of our patients. This explains the large difference that is found between the incidence and mortality of prostatic carcinoma. This phenomenon again depends on age. The effect of competing causes of death on the mortality of prostatic carcinoma can nicely be illustrated through the information depicted in table 3 of recent Dutch cancer statistics [6]. It can be seen that overall the incidence of prostatic carcinoma in The Netherlands during the years of 1975 – 76 was almost one-third higher than the mortality.

Table 3 Incidence and mortality of malignant neoplasms of the prostate by age, 1975 – 1976. (Figures are given per 100,000 of the average Dutch male population.)

Age	Incidence (absolute)	Incidence	Mortality
40 – 44	2	0.5	–
45 – 49	7	1.9	0.5
50 – 54	33	9.2	2.8
55 – 59	69	22.5	8.8
60 – 64	175	63.0	24.8
65 – 69	345	149.0	74.9
70 – 74	475	269.1	156.0
75 – 79	508	440.7	294.4
80 – 84	354	533.0	521.0
85 +	201	518.9	815.8
Total	2169	31.8	22.8

Centraal Bureau voor de Statistiek 1979

The natural course of each individual patient is obviously not identical to the general trend of the natural history of early prostatic cancer illustrated in this presentation. Still, treatment decisions have to be based on the scarse facts indicating the risks of the various lesions. The clinician is confronted with the difficult task to weigh the potential risks of the tumor in the individual case against the possible discomfort and side-effects resulting form treatment. This process is doomed to be successful only by approximation. The dilemma can only be solved by identifying morphological, functional or biochemical parameters that indicate clearly which tumor is likely to progress and which one is not. Until such information becomes available treatment decisions are bound to be determined by subjective criteria. Still, the information presented here is important for making daily decisions in this field.

The natural history of more extensive prostatic carcinoma is more easily described. It is characterized by progression to the metastatic state and independent of treatment roughly 50% of such patients will show progression to the hormone independent state within 2 years and will die within another year. The fate of our patients is determined by the step from hormone dependent to hormone independent growth. Research that is suitable to elucidate the mechanisms involved in this event must be given high priority.

References

[1] Akazaki, K., G. N. Stemmermann: Comparative study of latent carcinoma of the prostate among Japanese in Japan and Hawai. J. Nat. Cancer Inst. **50**, no. 5 (1973) 1137–1144.
[2] Blute, M. L., H. Zincke, G. M. Farrow: Long-term follow-up young patients with stage A adenocarcinoma of the prostate. J. Urol. **136** (1986) 840–843.
[3] Breslow, N., C. W. Chan, G. Dhom et al.: Latent carcinoma of prostate at autopsy in seven areas. Int. J. Cancer **20** (1977) 680–688.
[4] Byar, D. P., D. K. Corle (Veterans Administration Cooperative Urological Research Group): VACURG randomized trial of radical prostatectomy for stages I and II prostate cancer. Urology (Suppl.) **12**, No 4 (1981) 7–11.
[5] Cantrell, B. B., D. P. DeKlerk, J. C. Eggleston et al.: Pathological factors that influence prognosis in stage. A prostatic cancer: the influence of extent versus grade. J. Urol. **125** (1981) 516–520.
[6] Centraal Bureau voor de Statistiek: Kanker – morbiditeit en mortaliteit 1975/1976 (1981) 42–43.
[7] Epstein, J. I., G. Paull, J. C. Eggleston et al.: Prognosis of untreated stage A1 prostatic carcinoma: a study of 94 cases with extended follow-up. J. Urol. **136** (1986) 837–839.
[8] Kastendieck, H., E. Altenähr, H. Hüsselmann et al.: Carcinoma and dysplastic lesions of the prostate. Z. Krebsforsch. **88** (1976) 33–54.
[9] McNeal, J. E.: Origin and evolution of prostatic carcinoma. In: R. J. Ablin (ed.): Prostatic cancer, pp. 43–50. Marcel Dekker Inc., New York–Basel 1981.
[10] Whitmore, W. J., Jr.: Natural history and staging of prostate cancer. Urol. Clin. North Amer. **11** (1984) 205–220.
[11] Yamabe, H., F. J. W. ten Kate, M. P. W. Gallee et al.: Stage A prostatic cancer: a comparative study in Japan and the Netherlands. World J. Urol. **4** (1986) 136–140.

Pharmacological basis of androgen deprivation by various antiandrogens and their combination with LH-RH agonists

F. Neumann, M. F. El Etreby, U.-F. Habenicht, A. Radlmaier, K. Bormacher

Introduction

The basis of the therapy of hormone-dependent, metastatic carcinoma of the prostate is androgen deprivation, which can be achieved in two different ways: by reducing the available concentration of androgens – e.g. by means of orchiectomy or treatment with oestrogens, LH-RH agonists or inhibitors of steroid biosynthesis – or by inhibiting the effect of the available androgens at the cellular level, which is the mechanism of action of antiandrogens.

Although the peripheral mechanism of action of all antiandrogens is identical – i. e. competitive inhibition –, a distinction must be made between two completely different types of antiandrogens. On the one hand there are the so-called "pure" antiandrogens such as flutamide and anandron. In this context, the adjective "pure" means that these substances have only an antiandrogenic effect and no other endocrine properties. On the other hand, there are substances such as cyproterone acetate (CPA) and megestrol acetate, which display progestational properties as well. Because of their different spectrum of action, the two substance groups behave differently in vivo, a fact which has important implications for clinical use.

As regards the indication carcinoma of the prostate, two aspects in particular must be considered:

- advantages and disadvantages on use in monotherapy
- advantages and disadvantages on combined use with LH-RH analogues.

Monotherapy with antiandrogens

Because of the above-mentioned differences in the spectrum of action, the two types of antiandrogens affect the physiological regulatory axis – which keeps

New Developments in Biosciences 4

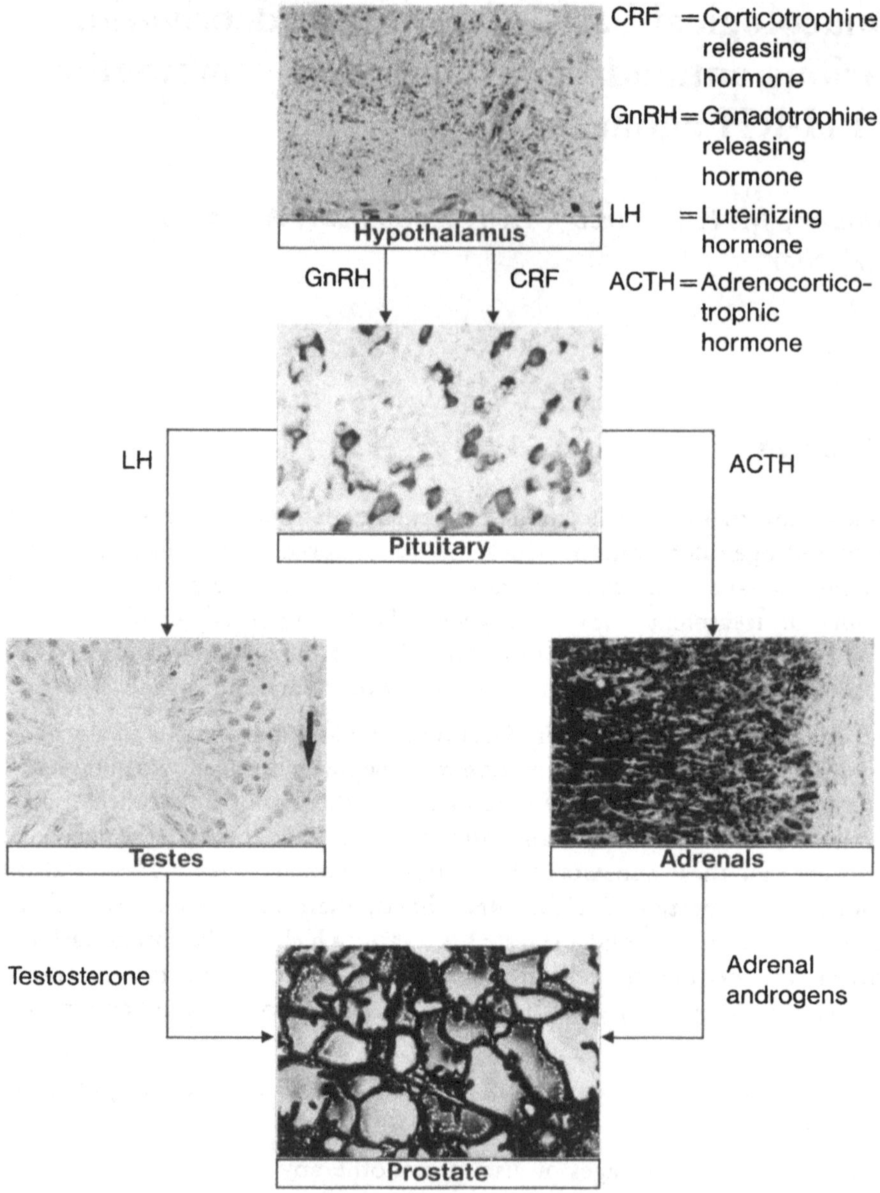

Fig. 1 Regulation of androgen production.

the concentration of testosterone within the normal range via the axis hypothalamus-pituitary-testes – in different ways.

The normal situation is shown in figure 1 for a better understanding. The hypothalamic releasing hormone LH-RH (luteinising hormone releasing hormone) stimulates the synthesis and release of the pituitary gonadotropins LH (luteinising hormone) and FSH (follicle-stimulating hormone). LH stimulates the biosynthesis of testosterone in the testes. In turn, the testosterone concentration in the blood influences the activity of the regulatory centre in the hypothalamus, i. e. more LH-RH is released when the testosterone concentration is low, whereas high testosterone concentrations inhibit the release of LH-RH. The phenomenon involved can therefore be regarded as a kybernetic system, similar to a thermostat.

Pure antiandrogens

The diagram in figure 2 shows how this kybernetic system reacts to pure antiandrogens, e. g. flutamide or anandron. These substances displace androgens from the central receptors at the hypothalamo-pituitary level where androgens exert their negative inhibitory effect. Consequently, an androgen deficit is simulated centrally which, in turn, triggers a counter-regulatory reaction involving the increased release of LH-RH and LH. This stimulates the biosynthesis of testosterone in the Leydig cells.

Permanent overstimulation leads to Leydig cell hyperplasia [27, 28, 36]. In animal experiments, definite histological changes have also been demonstrated in the pituitary (hyperplasia and hypertrophy of the gonadotropin-producing cells) [27, 36].

The intratesticular concentration of androgens increases dramatically under the influence of pure antiandrogens [36]. This explains why the disruptive effect of flutamide on spermatogenesis is, at the most, partial or only temporary (cf. fig. 3). As an example, rats were subfertile only at the start of treatment with flutamide – after 6 weeks, almost all the animals were fertile again even under very high doses [26, 32] (cf. tab. 1). Accordingly, flutamide is unable either at a testicular or at a hypothalamo-pituitary level to inhibit completely the effect of the increased biosynthesis of androgens. Because of this mechanism, the antiandrogenic effect

Table 1 Percentage of infertile male rats during treatment with flutamide administered in different dosages for various periods of time

Dose of Flutamide	Treatment period (weeks)			
(mg/d)	1	2	4	6
0.3	12	0	0	0
1.0	50	12	12	0
3.0	12	0	12	0
10.0	50	14	57	14

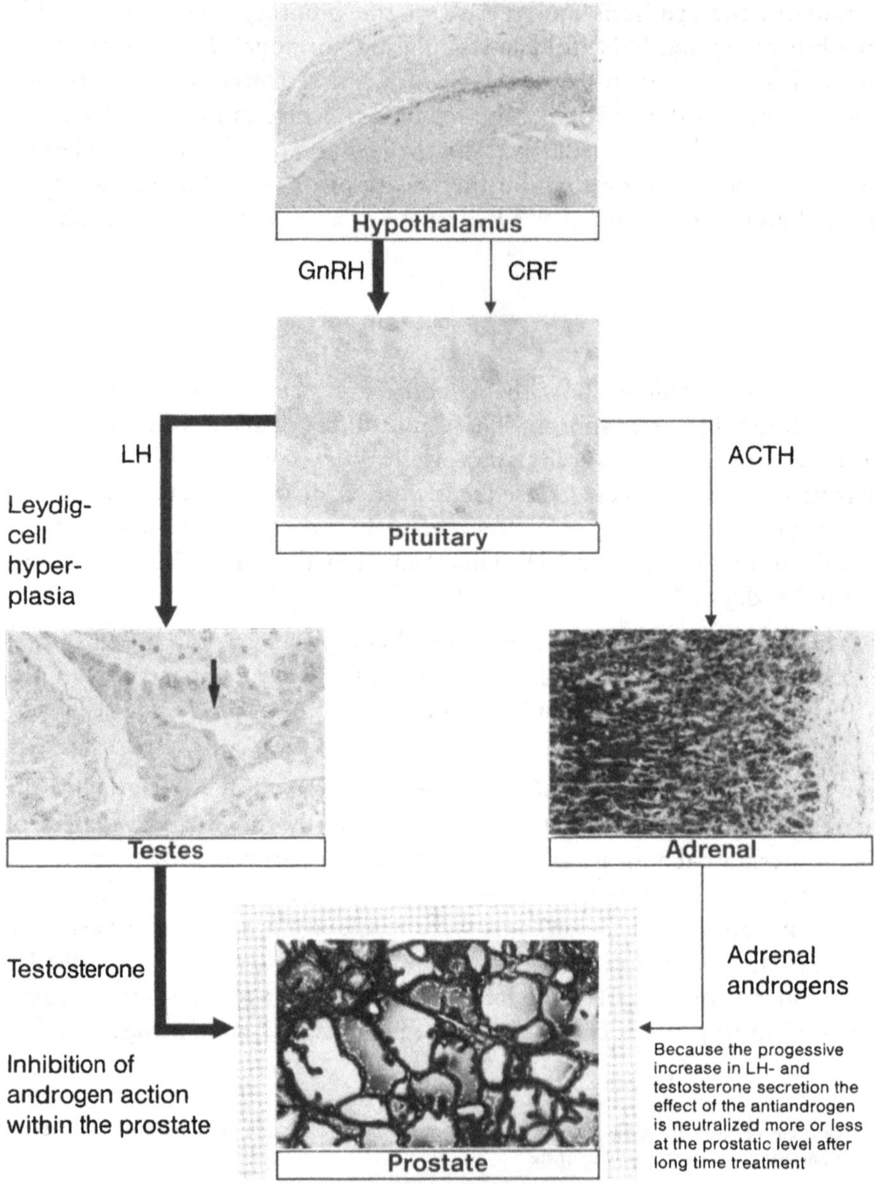

Fig. 2 Therapy with pure antiandrogens.

of a pure antiandrogen can, on prolonged administration, also be abrogated at the prostate, as has been demonstrated in an experiment in non-castrated rats [34] (cf. fig. 4).

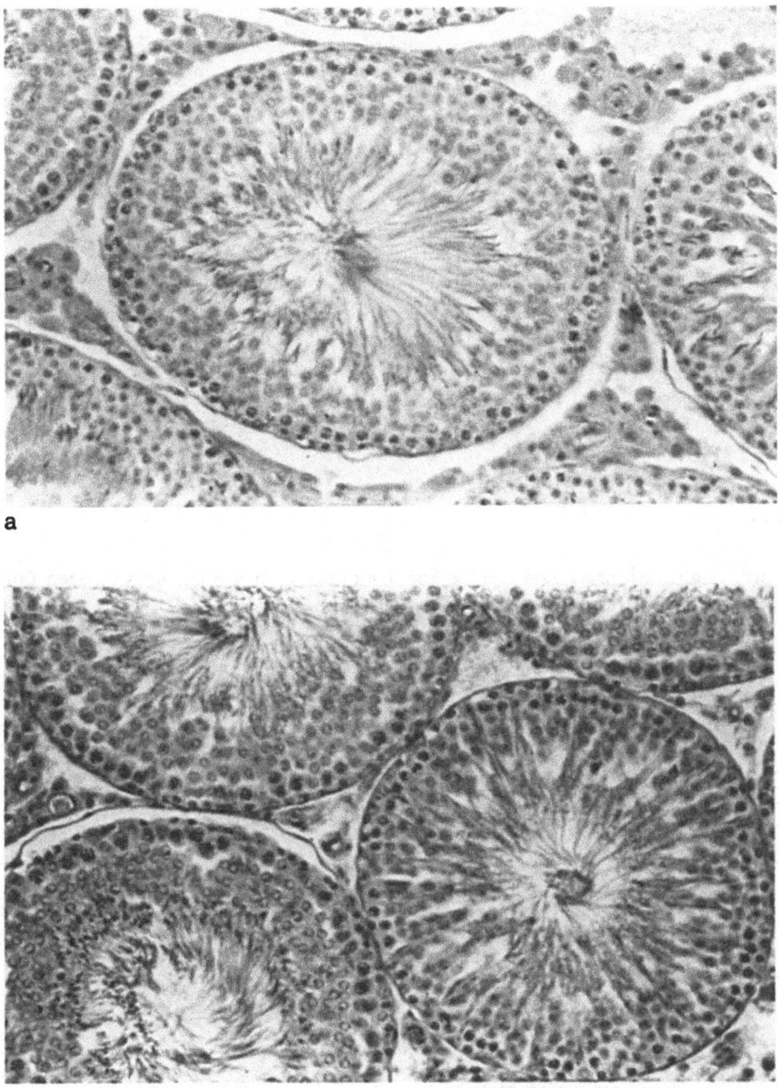

Fig. 3 Histology of rat testes (hematoxylin-eosin stain):
a) untreated control
b) treated with flutamide (10 mg/d) for 6 weeks.
Spermatogenesis remains unaffected.

The stimulation of androgen production by pure antiandrogens has also been observed in man: after 14 days' treatment of healthy men, LH in particular and, consecutively, also testosterone and estradiol were seen to increase [19](cf. fig. 5).

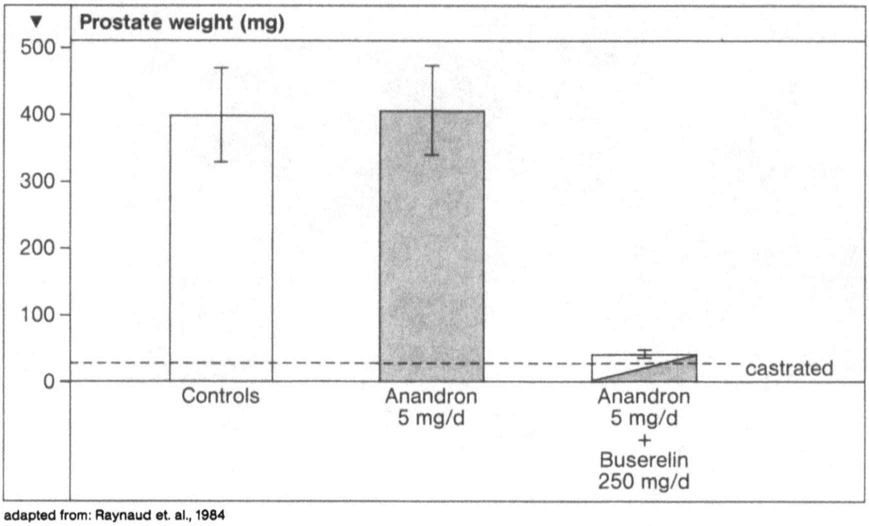

Fig. 4 Prostate weights of intact rats treated for 5 months with a pure antiandrogen (anandron) alone or in combination with an LHRH agonist (buserelin).

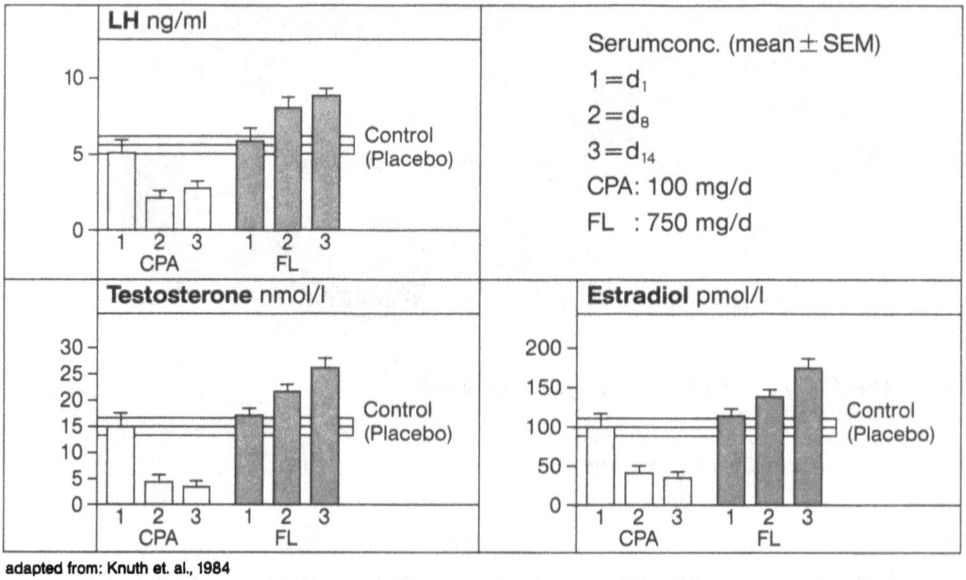

Fig. 5 Influence of cyproterone acetate (CPA) and flutamide (FL) on serum concentrations of LH, testosterone and estradiol in healthy males.

These examples show that, when administered alone, pure antiandrogens induce a counterregulatory increase of the testosterone concentration which can neutralise the effectiveness of the competitive inhibition, the decisive factor in which is the ratio of antiandrogen to testosterone. In other words, the possibility exists that the effect of a pure antiandrogen on androgen-dependent tissues will be more or less neutralised. Thus, the use of these substances as monotherapeutic agents in androgen-dependent carcinoma of the prostate entails an uncertainty factor which cannot be ignored.

The above-mentioned increase of estradiol results from the aromatisation of the increased amounts of testosterone. The increase of the estradiol concentration is accompanied by an increase of prolactin secretion, as has been demonstrated in transsexuals who had received anandron [13]. The frequent occurrence of gynaecomastia under therapy with pure antiandrogens is probably associated with the increase of estradiol and prolactin. In the case of the study with anandron in transsexuals, this “side effect” was desired.

Antiandrogens of the cyproterone acetate type

Antiandrogens of this type display not only pronounced antiandrogenic, but also potent progestational and, closely associated with this, antigonadotropic properties [25, 30] – i.e. they inhibit the secretion of gonadotropin and, hence, also the biosynthesis of testosterone. The influence of this type of antiandrogen on the hypothalamus-pituitary-testes axis is shown in the diagram in figure 6. As can be seen, androgen deprivation by cyproterone acetate is based on a dual mechanism of action:

- inhibition of the pituitary secretion of LH and, therefore, of the testicular biosynthesis of androgens,
- inhibition of the effect of the residual androgens (from the adrenals as well) by displacement from the receptors of the target organs.

As regards the central inhibitory antigonadotropic effect of cyproterone acetate, attention is drawn to the animal experiments [27, 36] and the pharmacological study in man already mentioned [19] (cf. fig. 5). In contrast to the situation under pure antiandrogens, the peripheral concentration of testosterone falls to well below the initial value under cyproterone acetate. This is also true for carcinoma patients [16] (cf. fig. 7).

Although the antigonadotropic effect and, hence, the inhibition of testosterone biosynthesis is not quite as pronounced as under oestrogen therapy, the additional antiandrogenic effect at the cellular level means that more effective androgen deprivation can be achieved at the target organ with CPA.

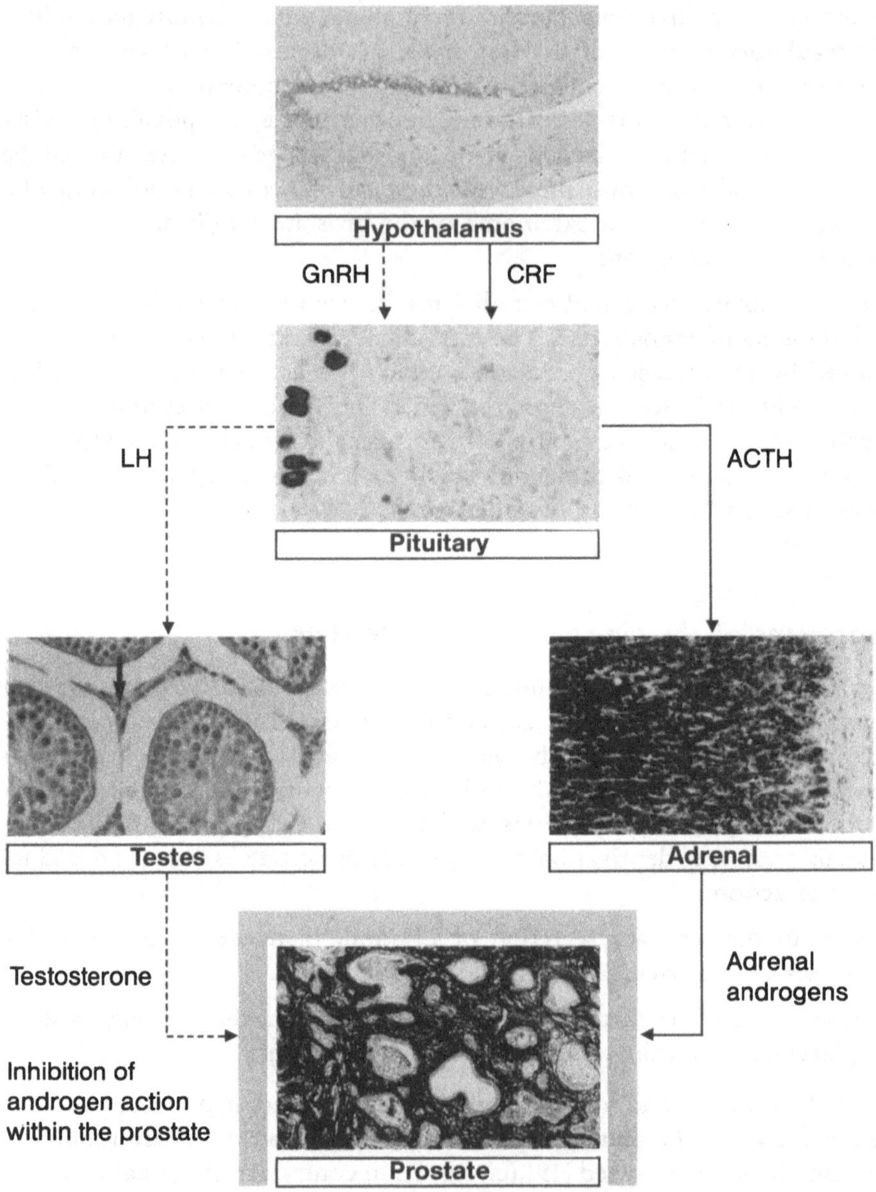

Fig. 6 Treatment with an antiandrogen of the cyproterone acetate type (additional antigonadotropic activity).

It has been shown in a large number of pharmacological studies that the effect of cyproterone acetate when given at high enough dosage is the same as that of surgical castration. This has been demonstrated, for example, by weighing the

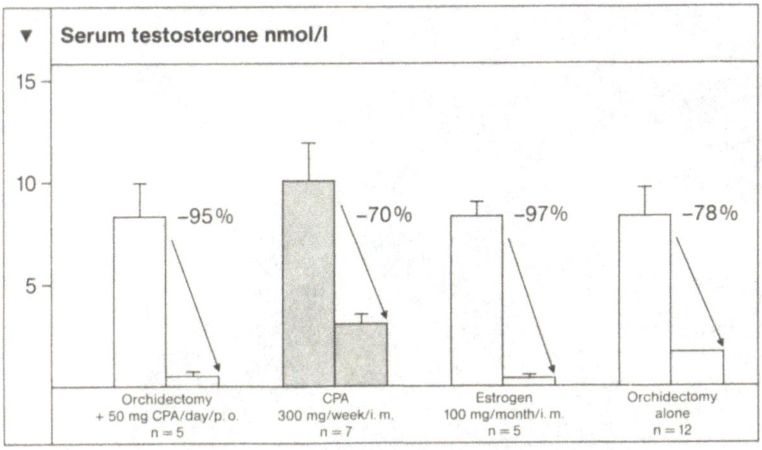

Fig. 7 Changes in peripheral testosterone concentration in patients with prostatic carcinoma treated with different forms of therapy for a period of 6 months.

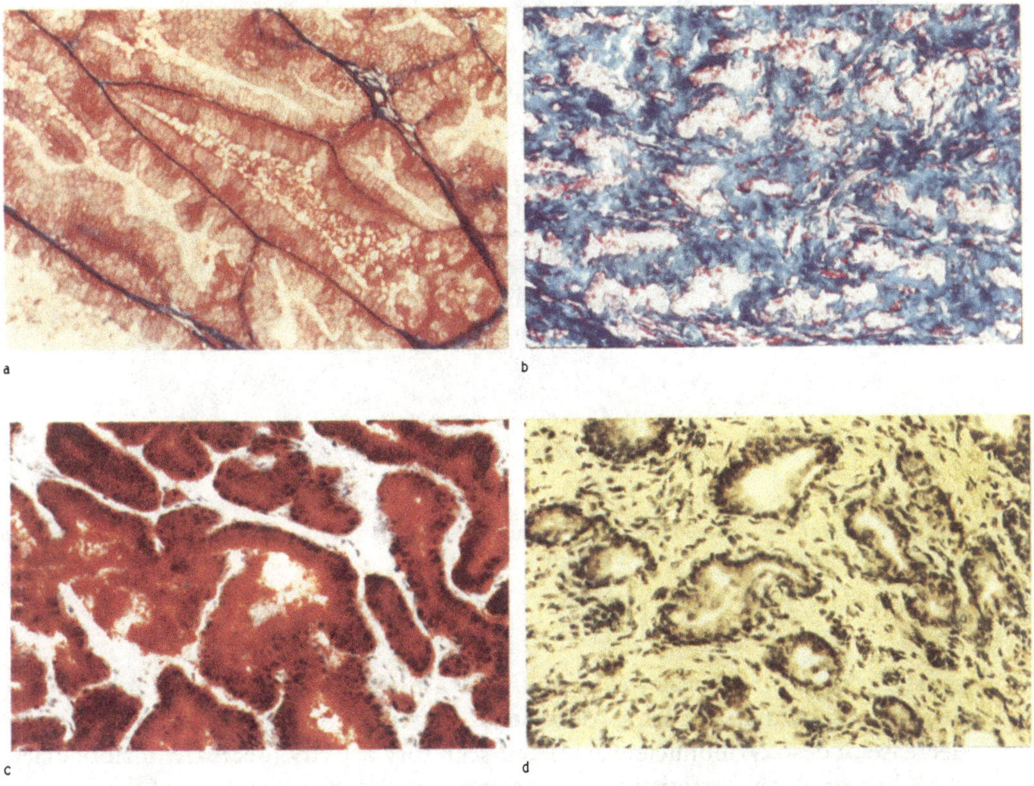

Fig. 8 Prostate histology of castrated dogs, treated with androstanediol alone or in combination with cyproterone acetate for 6 months.
(a + b: azan stain; c + d: acid phosphatase stain)
left: control; right: CPA 600 mg/weekly.

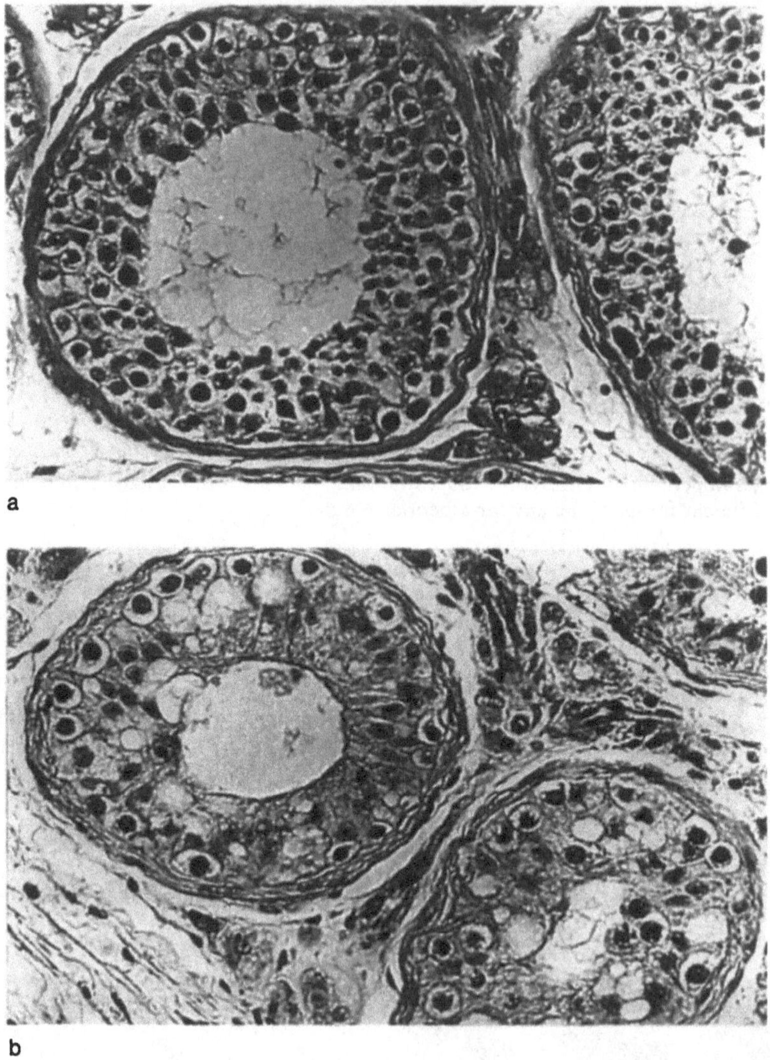

Fig. 9 Inhibition of spermatogenesis in a human male after about one year of treatment with cyproterone acetate (100 mg/d orally)
a) Control
b) Treated.

prostates of various species such as the rat, mouse and dog. Experiments in the dog have shown that both proliferative activity (a parameter of which is the decrease of desoxyribonucleic acid) and secretory activity (decrease of ribonucleic acid, loss of all characteristic enzymes and constituent substances of the prostate such as acid phosphatase, aminopeptidase and zinc) are reduced to castration levels [29, 30, 42, 43]. Figure 8 shows the histological changes of the prostate and the behavior of acid phosphatase in the dog after 6 months' administration of CPA. The complete atrophy of the epithelial part (fig. 8 b) and the complete loss of acid phosphatase (fig. 8 d) are clearly apparent.

The marked antiandrogenic effect also manifests itself at other androgen-dependent organs. For example, spermatogenesis is inhibited in both animals [31] and man [24, 37, 38]. Figure 9 b shows the testicular histology of a man treated with cyproterone acetate for about a year for suppression of drive. Distinct tubular atrophy and more or less complete inhibition of spermatogenesis can be observed even under 100 mg CPA/day. Meiosis no longer takes place [15]. It can be concluded from these and a number of other findings on the inhibition of androgen-dependent organs and functions that, in the man, a dose of about 200 mg CPA/day is sufficient to achieve an effect comparable to that of castration at the target organs for androgens [11, 32, 38, 39].

Combination of antiandrogens with LH-RH agonists

A new, pharmacological method of achieving androgen deprivation resembling the situation after orchiectomy is the use of LH-RH agonists. These substances are powerful stimulators of pituitary LH release. An initial phase lasting 2 to 3 weeks, during which the pituitary releases increased amounts of LH, is followed by the loss of pituitary LH-RH receptors and the cessation of LH secretion. As the LH concentration increases, so also does the concentration of testosterone. Thus, in the initial phase, testosterone increases to far above the pretreatment value. The conditions prevailing in the initial phase of monotherapy with an LH-RH agonist are therefore ideal for the growth of an androgen-dependent carcinoma.

It is well-documented that about 10 to 30% of patients treated with an LH-RH analogue alone display symptoms of tumour flare in the initial phase, a phenomenon which is undoubtedly attributable to the increased testicular biosynthesis of androgens in this phase [2, 6, 17, 33]. The main complaint of the patients is the increased metastatic pain. The tumour markers, e. g. acid phosphatase, also increase.

These undesired effects can be prevented by the administration of antiandrogens. But which type of antiandrogen is more suitable for the prophylaxis of tumour flare? A tentative answer is provided by some data from animal experiments. In a study in rats, an LH-RH analogue was combined with either flutamide or cyproterone acetate. LH and testosterone were then measured in the initial phase. It was found that the concentrations of LH and testosterone were increased after one week's treatment with an LH-RH agonist plus flutamide, but not after administration of cyproterone acetate in combination with the same agonist [14].

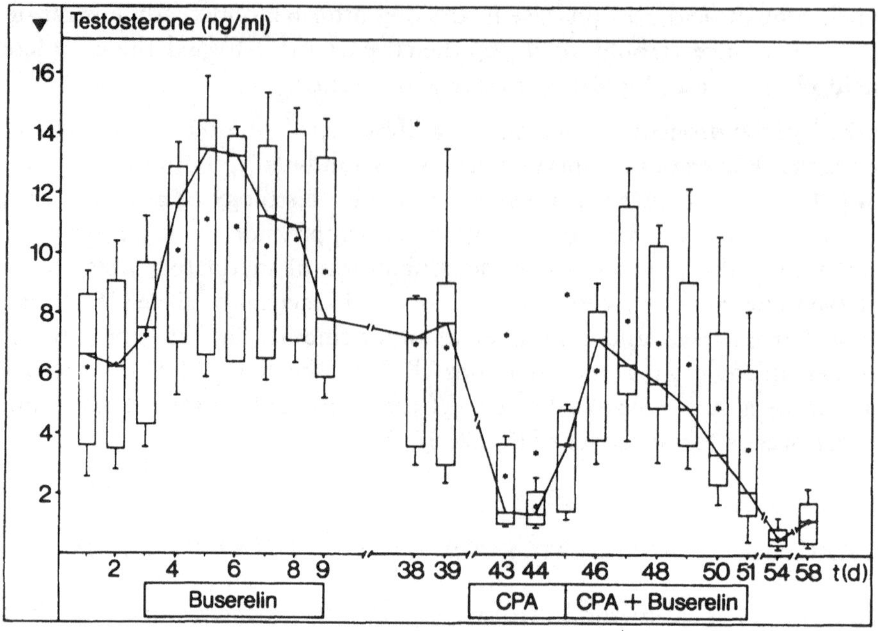

Fig. 10 Serum testosterone levels during the initial stimulatory phase in healthy men treated with an LHRH agonist alone or with additional cyproterone acetate-priming.

Studies in human volunteers have also shown that the initial increase of testosterone occurring under LH-RH agonists can be at least greatly reduced if the subject is treated beforehand with cyproterone acetate [14]. Some of the results of this study are shown in figure 10. The reduced testosterone values under the preceding treatment with CPA are increased only slightly by LH-RH agonist stimulation. This observation has been confirmed in patients. The initial increase of testosterone induced by LH-RH agonists and, hence, the flare phenomenon were avoided by preceding treatment with cyproterone acetate [5, 18, 41, 44].

The initial testosterone peak is not prevented under the combination of an LH-RH agonist with a pure antiandrogen. Because of the increased availability of testosterone, there is a risk that pure antiandrogens given in usual dosages are unable to suppress the effect of the androgens at the tumour cell to a sufficient degree. There are, in fact, observations of an initial increase of the tumour markers PAP and AP despite the additional administration of flutamide with an LH-RH agonist [4].

It can be concluded from this that, at least in the initial phase of therapy, antiandrogens with an antigonadotropic effect such as cyproterone acetate are preferable to pure antiandrogens for combining with an LH-RH agonist [35].

Some study groups recommend the combination of an LH-RH analogue with an antiandrogen for long-term use as well in order to bring about total androgen deprivation. This concept is based on the assumption that the adrenal androgens remaining after administration of LH-RH agonists (or castration) alone are sufficient to stimulate particularly androgen-sensitive tumour cell clones and, therefore, to induce progression [3, 21]. Thus, not only inhibition of the testicular androgens, but also elimination of the effect of the remaining adrenal androgens should be advocated.

A discussion of whether the additional blockade of adrenal androgens produces better therapeutic results is beyond the scope of this paper. Should this prove to be the case, however, the question arises which type of antiandrogen is more suitable for combining with an LH-RH agonist for long-term treatment.

In the late phase of LH-RH agonist therapy – after receptor down-regulation has occurred –, the counterregulatory increase of testosterone caused by pure antiandrogens administered alone fails to take place. Both types of antiandrogen are therefore equally suitable as regards the effectiveness of therapy.

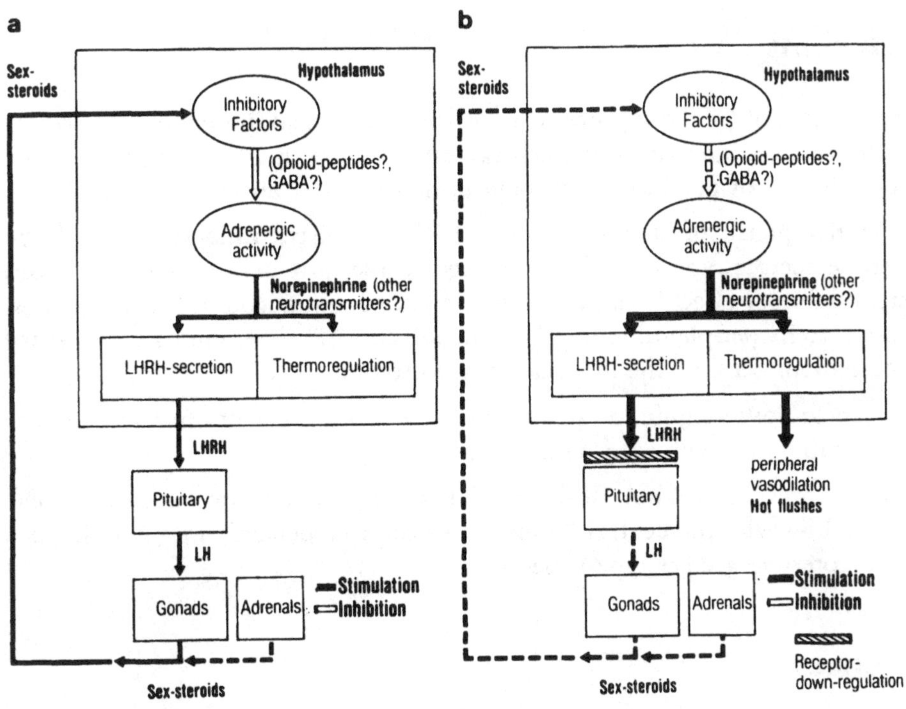

Fig. 11 Theoretical model of the neuroendocrine mechanism located in the hypothalamus which regulates LHRH-secretion and causes hot flushes:
a: Normal situation
b: Long-term therapy with LHRH agonists.

From the point of view regarding the side effects induced by LH-RH agonists, namely hot flushes, the central inhibitory activity of antiandrogens of the cyproterone acetate type offers an advantage. This can be explained in the following way: when an androgen deficit is brought about by LH-RH agonists or orchiectomy, the absence of inhibitory mechanisms leads to the stimulation of adrenergic neurones, i. e. to the increased release of norepinephrine. Norepinephrine, the neurotransmitter for LH-RH, not only stimulates the synthesis and release of LH-RH, but also affects central thermoregulation. The occurrence of hot flushes is therefore based on disturbances in this system in the sense of increased adrenergic activity (cf. fig. 11). The situation is comparable with that in postmenopausal women. The hot flushes can be prevented both by substances which suppress central adrenergic activity (clonidine) and by steroids with a central inhibitory component [cf. 1, 7, 10, 40]. Consequently, antiandrogens of the cyproterone acetate type are able to prevent the hot flushes occurring under LH-RH agonist therapy (as well as after castration) [8, 9, 12, 23]. This is not possible with antiandrogens without a central inhibitory effect such as flutamide and anandron [20, 22].

Conclusions

Only antiandrogens of the cyproterone acetate type with additional progestational and, therefore, antigonadotropic, central inhibitory properties are suitable for the monotherapy of prostatic carcinoma in non-orchiectomised patients.

In the initial phase of therapy with LH-RH agonists, antiandrogens of the cyproterone acetate type are to be preferred to the pure antiandrogens without a central inhibitory effect because of their additional antigonadotropic properties. In addition to its peripheral antiandrogenic effect, CPA also inhibits the primary cause of tumour flare – the increase of testosterone.

After receptor down-regulation has taken place, both types of antiandrogen are equally suitable for combining with an LH-RH agonist.

In order to prevent the hot flushes which occur on deprivation of testicular androgens, however, the central inhibitory effect inherent only in antiandrogens of the cyproterone acetate type is necessary.

References

[1] Abdalla, H. I.: Pathophysiology of hot flushes. Obstet. Gynecol. Surv. 40 (1985) 338–343.

[2] Ahmed, S. R., J. Grant, S. M. Shalet et al.: Preliminary report on use of depot formulation of LHRH analogue ICI 118630 (Zoladex) in patients with prostatic cancer. Brit. Med. J. 290 (1985) 185–187.

[3] Allen, J. M., D. J. Kerle, H. Ware et al.: Combined treatment with ketoconazole and LHRH analogue: a novel approach to resistant progressive prostatic cancer. Brit. Med. J. **287** (1983) 1766.

[4] Aulitzky, W., J. Frick, H. Joos et al.: Inhibition of LHRH-analogue induced testosterone surge by blockade of androgen receptors. 82nd meeting American Urological Association (AUA) 1987.

[5] Boccon-Gibod, L., M. H. Laudat, M. A. Dugue: Cyproterone acetate lead-in prevents initial rise of serum testosterone induced by LHRH analogs in the treatment of metastatic carcinoma of the prostate. Eur. Urol. 12 (1986) 400–402.

[6] Boumier, P., A.-C. Koeger, J. P. Camus: Aggraviation dramatique d'un cancer prostatique au début d'un traitement par un agoniste de la gonadoréline. Presse méd. **14** (1984) 1200–1201.

[7] Casper, R. F., S. S. C. Yen: Neuroendocrinology of menopausal flushes: an hypothesis of flush mechanism. Clin. Endocrinol. 22 (1985) 293–312.

[8] Claes, H., L. Vanderbussche, R. L. Vereecken: Treatment of advanced carcinoma of the prostate by LHRH agonists. 7th Congr. Europ. Assoc. Urol., Budapest/Hungary 1986.

[9] Eaton, A. C., N. McGuire: Cyproterone acetate in treatment of post-orchidectomy hot flushes. Lancet **8363** (1983) 1336–1337.

[10] Frödin, T., G. Alund, E. Varenhorst: Measurement of skin blood-flow and water evaporation as a means of objectively assessing hot flushes after orchidectomy in patients with prostatic cancer. Prostate 7 (1985) 203–208.

[11] Giese, H., W. F. J. Krause, H. Schmidt: Sexualhormone in Beziehung zur Sexualität. Forum der Psychiatrie **20** (1968) 189–200.

[12] Gingell, J. C.: Does orchidectomy cause excessive sweating? Brit. Med. J. **288** (1984) 709.

[13] Gooren, L., T. Spinder, J. J. Spijkstra et al.: Sex steroids and pulsatile LH release in men. Studies in estrogen-treated agonadal subjects and eugonadal subjects treated with a novel nonsteroidal antiandrogen. J. Clin. Endocrinol. Metab. **64** (1987) 763–770.

[14] Habenicht, U.-F., E. Witthaus, F. Neumann: Antiandrogene und LHRH-Agonisten: Endokrinologie in der Initialphase ihrer Anwendung. Akt. Urol. 17 (1986) 10–16.

[15] Horn, H. J.: Administration of antiandrogens in hypersexuality and sexual deviations. In: O. Eichler, A. Farah, H. Herken et al. (eds): Androgens II and antiandrogens, Chap. 8, pp. 543–562. Springer, Berlin, Heidelberg, New York 1974.

[16] Jacobi, G. H., U. Tunn, Th. Senge: Clinical experience with cyproterone acetate for palliation of inoperable prostate cancer. In: G. H. Jacobi, R. Hohenfellner (eds): Prostate cancer, Vol. 3, pp. 305–319. Williams & Wilkins, Baltimore, London 1982.

[17] Kahan, A., F. Delrieu, B. Amor et al.: Disease flare induced by D-Trp-6-LHRH analogue in patients with metastatic prostatic cancer. Lancet **8383** (1984) 971–972.

[18] Klign, J. G. M., H. J. de Voogt, F. H. Schröder et al.: Combined treatment with buserelin and cyproterone acetate in metastatic prostatic carcinoma. Lancet **8453** (1985) 493.

[19] Knuth, U. A., R. Hano, E. Nieschlag: Effect of flutamide or cyproterone acetate on pituitary and testicular hormones in normal men. J. Clin. Endocrinol. Metab. **59** (1984) 963–969.

[20] Labrie, F., A. Dupont, A. Belanger et al.: New approach in the treatment of prostate cancer: complete instead of partial withdrawal of androgens. Prostate **4** (1983) 579–594.

[21] Labrie, F., A. Dupont, A. Belanger et al.: New hormonal treatment in cancer of the prostate: combined administration of an LHRH agonist and an antiandrogen. J. steroid Biochem. **19** (1983) 999–1007.

[22] Migliari, R., R. M. Scarpa, S. Balzano et al.: Combined treatment with flutamide and buserelin in advanced prostate cancer. 1 year of experience. J. Endocrinol. Invest. **10** (Suppl. 2) (1987) 58.

[23] Moon, T. D.: Cyproterone acetate for treatment of hot flushes after orchiectomy. J. Urol. **134** (1985) 155–156.

[24] Morse, H. C., D. R. Leach, M. J. Rowley et al.: Effect of cyproterone acetate on sperm concentration, seminal fluid volume, testicular cytology and levels of plasma and urinary ICSH, FSH and testosterone in normal men. J. Reprod. Fert. 32 (1973) 365–378.

[25] Neumann, F.: Pharmacology and clinical uses of cyproterone acetate. In: B. J. A. Furr, A. Wakeling (eds): Pharmacology and clinical uses of inhibitors of hormone secretion and action, Chap. 7, pp. 132–159. Baillière Tindall, London, Philadelphia, Toronto 1987.

[26] Neumann, F., M. F. El Etreby, U.-F. Habenicht et al.: Möglichkeiten des Androgenentzugs und der totalen Blockade. In: R. Nagel (ed): Konservative Therapie des Prostatakarzinoms, pp. 61 – 86. Springer, Berlin, Heidelberg, New York, London, Paris, Tokyo 1987.

[27] Neumann, F., K.-J. Gräf, S. H. Hasan et al.: Central actions of antiandrogens. In: L. Martini, M. Motta (eds): Androgens and antiandrogens, pp. 163 – 177. Raven, New York 1977.

[28] Neumann, F., U.-F. Habenicht, A. Schacher: Antiandrogens and target cell response – different in vivo effects of cyproterone acetate, flutamide and cyproterone. In: K. W. McKerns, A. Aakvaag, V. Hansson (eds): Regulation of target cell responsiveness, Vol. II, pp. 489 – 527. Plenum, New York 1984.

[29] Neumann, F., M. Hümpel, Th. Senge et al.: Cyproterone acetate – biochemical and biological basis for treatment of prostatic cancer. In: G. H. Jacobi, R. Hohenfellner (eds): Prostate cancer, Vol. 3, pp. 269 – 303. Williams & Wilkins, Baltimore, London 1982.

[30] Neumann, F., G. H. Jacobi: Antiandrogens in tumour therapy. In: B. J. A. Furr (ed): Clinics in oncology, Vol. 1, Chap. 3, pp. 41 – 64. W. B. Saunders, London, Philadelphia 1982.

[31] Neumann, F., B. Schenck: Antiandrogens: Basic concepts and clinical trials. In: G. R. Cunningham, W.-B. Schill, E. S. E. Hafez (eds): Regulation of male fertility, Vol. 5, pp. 93 – 104. Martinus Nijhoff, The Hague, Boston, London 1980.

[32] Ott, F., H. Hoffet: Beeinflussung von Libido, Potenz und Hodenfunktion durch Antiandrogene. Schweiz. Med. Wschr. 98 (1968) 1812 – 1815.

[33] Parmar, H., S. L. Lightman, L. Allen et al.: Randomised controlled study of orchidectomy vs. long-acting D-Trp-6-LHRH microcapsules in advanced prostatic carcinoma. Lancet **8466** (1985) 1201 – 1205.

[34] Raynaud, J. P., C. Bonne, M. Moguilewsky et al.: The pure antiandrogen RU 23 908 (Anandron®), a candidate of choice for the combined antihormonal treatment of prostatic cancer: a review. Prostate 5 (1984) 299 – 311.

[35] Sandow, J.: Discussion remark. In: Excerpta Medica for Hoechst AG (ed): Chap.: Combining buserelin with antiandrogens – against flare and in the long term. The Releaser **1** (1986) 14 – 15.

[36] Schacher, A., M. F. El Etreby, F. Neumann: Einfluß von Cyproteronacetat, Flutamid und Spironolacton auf die Achse Hypothalamus – Hypophyse – Hoden bei Ratten. Akt. Urol. 15 (1984) 218 – 225.

[37] Schulze, W.: Licht- und elektronenmikroskopische Studien an den A-Spermatogonien von Männern mit intakter Spermatogenese und bei Patienten nach Behandlung mit Antiandrogenen. andrologia 10 (1978) 307 – 320.

[38] Städtler, F., H. J. Horn: Veränderungen an menschlichen Hoden während einer Antiandrogen-Behandlung. Dtsch. med. Wschr. **98** (1973) 1013 – 1019.

[39] Städtler, F., H. Zaun: Vergleichende Auswertung von Hodenbiopsie- und Haarwurzel-Statusbefunden unter antiandrogener Behandlung. andrologia 6 (1974) 303 – 314.

[40] Steinfeld, A. D., Ch. Reinhardt: Male climacteric after orchiectomy in patient with prostatic cancer. Urology **16** (1980) 620 – 622.

[41] Svensson, M., E. Varenhorst, B. Kagedal: Initial administration of cyproterone acetate to prevent the rise of testosterone concentration during treatment with an LHRH agonist in prostatic cancer. Anticancer Res. 6 (1986) 379.

[42] Tunn, U., Th. Senge, B. Schenck et al.: Biochemical and histological studies on prostates in castrated dogs after treatment with androstanediol, oestradiol and cyproterone acetate. Acta Endocrinol. (Copenh.) 91 (1979) 373 – 384.

[43] Tunn, U., Th. Senge, B. Schenck et al.: Effects of cyproterone acetate on experimentally induced canine prostatic hyperplasia. A morphological and histochemical study. Urol. Int. 35 (1980) 125 – 140.

[44] Urwin, G. H., J. L. Williams, J. A. Kanis: Antiandrogens attenuate testosterone 'flare' following Zoladex depot LHRH analogue in patients with prostatic cancer. 7th Congr. Europ. Assoc. Urol., Budapest/Hungary 1986.

III Clinics

Evaluation of different endocrine approaches in the treatment of prostatic carcinoma

A. O. Turkes, W. B. Peeling, D. W. Wilson, K. Griffiths

Introduction

Our understanding of the endocrine factors that may be concerned in the control of prostatic growth and function has increased immensely over the past few years and the role of prolactin or growth hormone, or the influence of the adrenal C_{19}-steroid secretion, on prostatic function illustrate certain relationships that generate particular interest [17 – 19]. Despite this, it is evident that the prostate gland is primarily dependent upon testosterone, of which 90 – 95% is secreted by the testis (fig. 1) and the cornerstone of our treatment of prostatic cancer is that since the cancer retains some degree of hormone-dependence similar to the normal gland, primary therapy must be based on the removal of this testicular source of androgen. It was the experimental studies of Huggins and his colleagues [21 – 23] in the early 1940's which established the scientific basis for the treatment of advanced prostatic cancer and orchidectomy, or treatment with the then new, synthetic oestrogen diethylstilboestrol (DES) was shown to relieve the symptoms and improve the general well-being of men with the disease [23]. Orchidectomy or treatment with DES have therefore been the mainstay of treatment for advanced prostatic cancer for these ensuing four decades. Orchidectomy, although a simple, effective procedure, is however permanent, mutilating and generally distasteful to most males. It has been generally accepted that DES provides an alternative inexpensive and relatively successful form of therapy for the management of the disease, exercising its effect on the cancer indirectly by the suppression of pituitary release of luteinizing hormone (LH) thereby decreasing the synthesis and secretion of testicular testosterone.

Metastatic carcinoma of the prostate responds to this primary endocrine therapy with approximately 70% of patients experiencing symptomatic relief [39, 43] although relapse generally occurs within 1 – 2 years [27, 58] and the median survival is then 6 months. Disease progression is considered a result of the inexorable growth of the hormone-independent, autonomous cancer cells. The early hope therefore that the endocrine approach to treatment heralded a real

New Developments in Biosciences 4

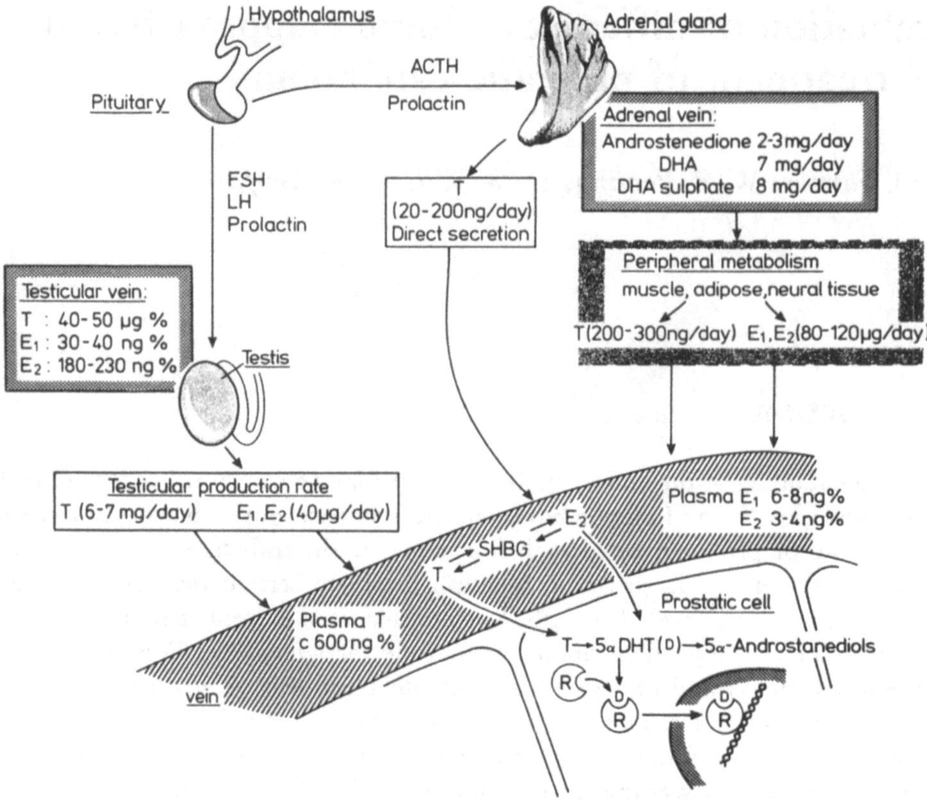

Fig. 1 Schematic representation of some of the steroid and peptide hormones that are concerned with the regulation of prostatic function. DHA, dehydroepiandrosterone; 5α-DHT, 5α-dihydrotestosterone; SHBG, sex hormone binding globulin; T, testosterone; E_1, oestrone; E_2, oestradiol-17β; R_1, specific intracellular receptor.

cure has been dispelled through succeeding years. Palliation was possible and there can be improvement in the quality of life, but investigators continue to search for new initiatives that may benefit the patient.

Primary endocrine therapy

Bilateral orchidectomy is therefore a simple surgical procedure to remove the primary source of testosterone decreasing the concentration of the androgen in plasma to 'castrate level' of 2 nmol/L (fig. 2). Residual plasma testosterone is of adrenal origin [17, 19]. DES treatment in its currently conventional dose of 1 mg (t. d. s.) reduces plasma terstosterone concentrations to the same 'castrate level'.

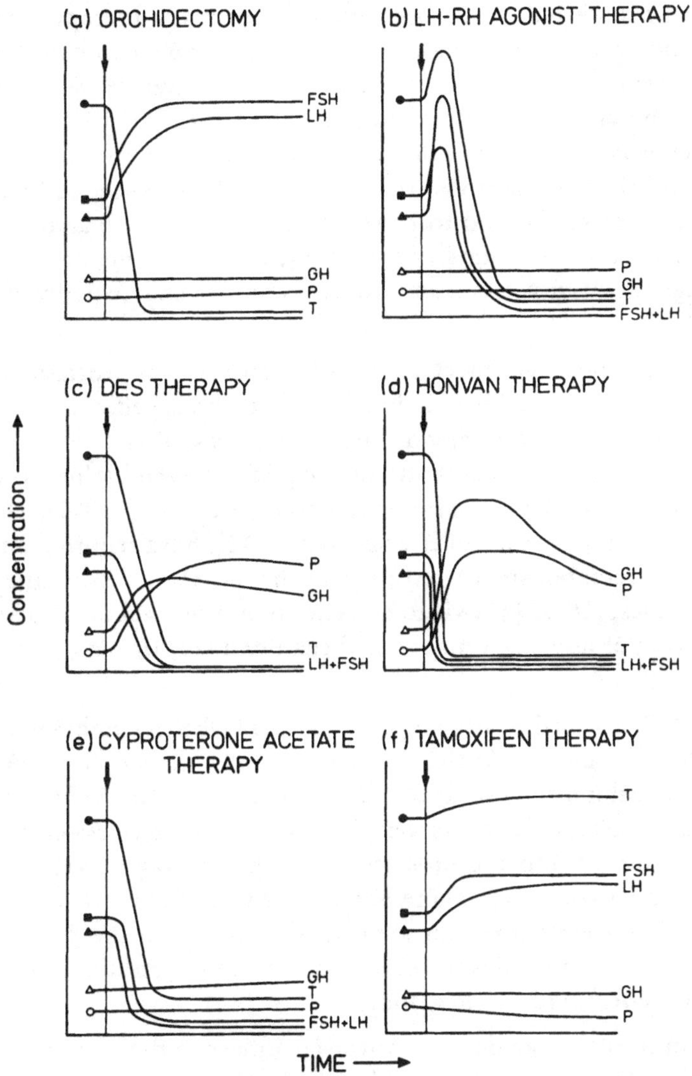

Fig. 2 Schematic representation of the changes in the concentration of plasma hormones during endocrine therapy for prostatic cancer. Concentrations are represented as arbitrary units. Data from the Tenovus Institute for Cancer Research.

Few drugs other than DES have gained universal acceptance. The long-acting intramuscular polyoestradiol phosphate (Estradurin) is popular in Scandinavia but only weakly suppresses LH secretion [25, 32] and Premarin (2.5 mg t. d. s.) a mixture of conjugated equine oestrogens or ethinyloestradiol (0.15 – 1.0 mg/day) have generally been considered less effective than DES and more expensive.

Various progestational steroids have been used for primary therapy including medroxyprogesterone acetate (Provera), hydroxyprogesterone caproate (Delalutin), cyproterone acetate (Cyprostat) and chlormadinone acetate. Some, would certainly consider the clinical results of promise [14], but it must be accepted that, apart from cyproterone acetate, their effectiveness or clinical value has not been critically established by rigorous, randomised trials. Consequently, at present, these drugs cannot yet be said to have a major role in the management of advanced prostatic cancer. In contrast, cyproterone acetate having an additional strong anti-androgenic activity, has been proven to be clinically equally effective as DES [38 b, 55 b].

There is evidence of a possible direct action of oestrogen on prostatic growth and function [12, 17, 38 a, 46]. Little is known about the specific physiological role of oestrogens in the prostate gland, but the impression is that a dynamic relationship exists between androgens and oestrogens with the biological effects of one being influenced by the presence of the other. Farnsworth [12], Danutra and her colleagues [9] and various other groups [3, 9, 12], have reported an effect of oestrogen on the metabolism of testosterone by prostatic tissue and more earlier, classical studies, [16, 21] provided evidence of a direct action of oestrogen on prostatic secretion of androgen-maintained castrated [21] or hypophysectomised dogs [16].

Nesbit and Baum [37] claimed nearly 40 years ago that DES in combination with orchidectomy offered a more effective form of therapy than either procedure alone. The rationale behind the use of DES-diphoshate (Honvan, Stilphostrol) in doses often exceeding 200 mg daily was that the free, presumably active, cytotoxic DES was released directly into the prostate cancer by the high levels of phosphatase present in the tissue [51]. There appears little evidence to support this concept [1], DES-diphosphate does not seem to accumulate in the prostate and the high levels of DES in the plasma after Honvan administration could well exercise a cytotoxic effect within the gland.

The use of Honvan in such high doses is however subject to the same difficulties inherent in the use of DES which were highlighted by the report of the VACURG (Veterans Administration Cooperative Urological Research Group) investigations [2, 7, 35]. The cardiovascular problems caused by the clinical use of DES have elicited considerable concern and the other reported side-effects, including feminisation, decreased libido, impotence, azoospermia, nausea and gastric disturbances have long been associated with DES therapy. The side-effects are however dose-related and are minimal if 1 mg DES is administered daily, although in the United Kingdom, this dose is not considered [45] sufficient to control testicular function and 1 mg t. d. s. is the accepted regime; certainly 1 mg t. d. s. is just as effective as Honvan in larger doses in reducing the concentration of testosterone in plasma to 'castrate' levels (fig. 2).

The marked elevation in the plasma concentrations of prolactin and growth hormone observed after larger doses of oestrogen (fig. 2) may well be considered a contra-indication in view of the suggested influence of prolactin on adrenal C_{19}-steroid synthesis [19, 20] and on the uptake of androgens and their metabolism by prostate tissue. Honvan's use has generally fallen from favour, although it may have some value administered intravenously when a rapid response is required for patients with severe metastatic bone pain [39].

The concept of drug targetting was incorporated into the research programme of the Tenovus Institute in the late 1960's on the basis that in cancer chemotherapy, it is important to localise the action of the drug primarily within the tumour. In association with the late Dr. Arthur Walpole, (I. C. I., U. K.), two nitrogen mustard derivatives, of DES (I. C. I. 85966) and of tamoxifen (I. C. I., 79792), were prepared and their biological effects studied [18]. The introduction of estramustine phosphate (Estracyt), with the alkylating agent, nor-nitrogen mustard attached as a carbamate via C-3 of oestradiol-17β, was equally of interest. Despite being oestrogenic and cytotoxic, Estracyt has never been as universally accepted as might have been expected. Generally results indicate that as primary therapy, Estracyt is only as effective as conventional oestrogen treatment [24, 26, 31, 55 a], although it was reported [11] that approximately 40% of patients, refractory to orchidectomy or oestrogen treatment, responded to the drug, an effect which requires substantiation by a phase III randomised clinical trial. Whatever its chemotherapeutic effect, part of its clinical action will be endocrine orientated since the concentration of plasma oestradiol-17β is significantly elevated in patients treated with Estracyt [18].

Secondary endocrine therapy

It is stated that of the patients who relapse after primary therapy, only a small proportion will respond to further endocrine treatment [5], especially orchidectomy after prolonged oestrogen therapy, although hypophysectomy seems to offer worthwhile palliation of pain without affecting survival [13]. Generally the concentration of testosterone in the plasma of patients on long-term DES therapy would not change after administration of LH-RH and the testosterone concentration has been shown to remain at the 'castrate' level [19, 28]. In one particular study [28] one of six patients studied on long-term oestrogen therapy had relatively high levels of plasma testosterone and responded to i. v. LH-RH administration. A daily regimen of 3 mg DES was insufficient to control testicular secretion of testosterone. Failure to respond to treatment was not due to hormone-independent cancer but in this patient, to inadequate dosage with DES. Although orchidectomy as secondary endocrine therapy is now recognised as having little value [50], removal of the testes in this particular patient could well have been beneficial.

There is little doubt that the 'residual' testosterone in the plasma of castrated patients or those on oestrogen therapy, is of adrenal origin [8, 41] although relapse, or disease progression is rarely associated with a secondary rise in the testosterone level [20]. Whether the adrenal androgens do play a role in maintaining the growth of hormone-dependent cancer cells is still being questioned. It was this concern that the adrenal androgens continued to sustain prostate cancer that provoked Huggins to adrenalectomise his patients in order to manage the disease although reports of the results of this form of therapy are not encouraging [4].

Anti-androgens, including flutamide [48, 49] and cyproterone acetate [47] have also been used to treat relapsed patients on the basis that they would restrain the adrenal androgen action at the target organ. Response to this secondary therapy is reported in a smaller proportion of patients. The potential of progestational steroids has been assessed by Geller [14, 15]. These steroids both inhibit LH secretion and influence the effect of 5α-dihydrotestosterone in the prostate, although their clinical value has again not been established by rigorous clinical trials. Similarly the potential of aminoglutethimide for secondary endocrine therapy has been assessed [10, 36], a drug which inhibits adrenal C_{19}-steroid synthesis.

To many urologists however, disease progression is considered to relate to the growth of clones of hormone-independent cancer cells and it may be that selected cytotoxic therapy may be necessary for the more successful management of the relapsed patient, or the patient who fails primary endocrine therapy.

LH-RH analogues

The concern that followed the reports [7] of the potential cardiovascular problems associated with oestrogen therapy has tended to evoke a reversion to the use of bilateral orchidectomy for the management of disseminated prostatic cancer, or in the United Kingdom, to reconsider subcapsular orchidectomy. It is certainly the opinion of many that orchidectomy is the yardstick against which all other forms of endocrine therapy should be assessed. Subcapsular orchidectomy, introduced in 1942 [44], fell into disrepute when it was subsequently reported [34] that Leydig cells remained on the tunica albuginea and the vascular hilum of the testes after the operation. Recent studies [6, 54] indicate that the operation is as effective as total orchidectomy and human chorionic gonadotrophin administration to treated patients failed to elevate plasma concentrations of testosterone.

Current interest however centres on the clinical use of the LH-RH analogues, in particular on the relationship between adrenal androgens and prostatic cancer and the potential of the more aggressive approach to primary endocrine therapy, the 'complete androgen blockade' [29, 30], the simultaneous treatment with an LH-RH analogue, or antitesticular therapy, and an anti-androgen.

Preliminary investigations from the Tenovus Institute indicated [33] that atrophy of the gonads resulted from the pharmacological doses of the LH-RH analogue, I. C. I. 118630 (Zoladex, D-Ser(Bu^t)^{6}Azgly^{10}-LH-RH, I. C. I. Pharmaceuticals, Macclesfield, Cheshire, U. K.). Low doses mimic the physiological action of LH-RH, stimulating the pituitary secretion of gonadotrophins whereas the continuous administration of pharmacological amounts produced the paradoxical antigonadal effect. Early clinical studies with the Yorkshire Prostate Group [56] established the effectiveness of Zoladex in reducing plasma testosterone levels and phase II trials in South Wales [57] using a slow-release (depot) formulation [19, 41] clearly demonstrated the efficacy of the preparation in producing a medical castration. Depot Zoladex is administered as a single monthly injection. The decapeptide is incorporated into a 50 : 50 lactide : glycolide copolymer in the form of a small cylindrical rod which is injected into the subcutaneous tissue of the anterior abdominal wall. A study [57] in which patients were randomised to one of three doses of depot Zoladex, 3.6, 1.8 or 0.9 mg over 4 weeks indicated that the plasma testosterone concentrations fell to 'castrate' levels within 15 – 22 days, with the 3.6 mg dose being marginally more effective, and complete pituitary desensitisation following the second and third subsequent injections (fig. 3).

This very practical, innovative means of administering the LH-RH analogue is clinically most effective and a phase III randomised clinical trial, involving 18 urological clinics of the British Prostate Study Group and coordinated by the Tenovus Institute [40, 52, 53] has recently finished recruitment of 358 patients over a 15-month period. The long term administration of depot Zoladex, 3.6 g monthly, was shown to be clinically as effective as orchidectomy for the clinical management of metastatic prostatic cancer.

In association with clinical colleagues of the British Prostate Study Group, and with Schering, U. K., the Tenovus Institute is participating in a new randomised clinical trial of Zoladex and the anti-androgen, cyproterone acetate against Zoladex alone and also against cyproterone acetate alone to assess further the value of the combined therapy for the management of the disease. The clinical value of the more aggressive endocrine approach, with therapy directed to the suppression of testicular secretion of testosterone and the blockage of residual androgen at the level of the target prostate cancer cell is currently being assessed in many other centres around the world and the results are awaited with interest. It must be emphasised however that a large proportion of patients who present with metastatic carcinoma of the prostate fail to respond to endocrine therapy

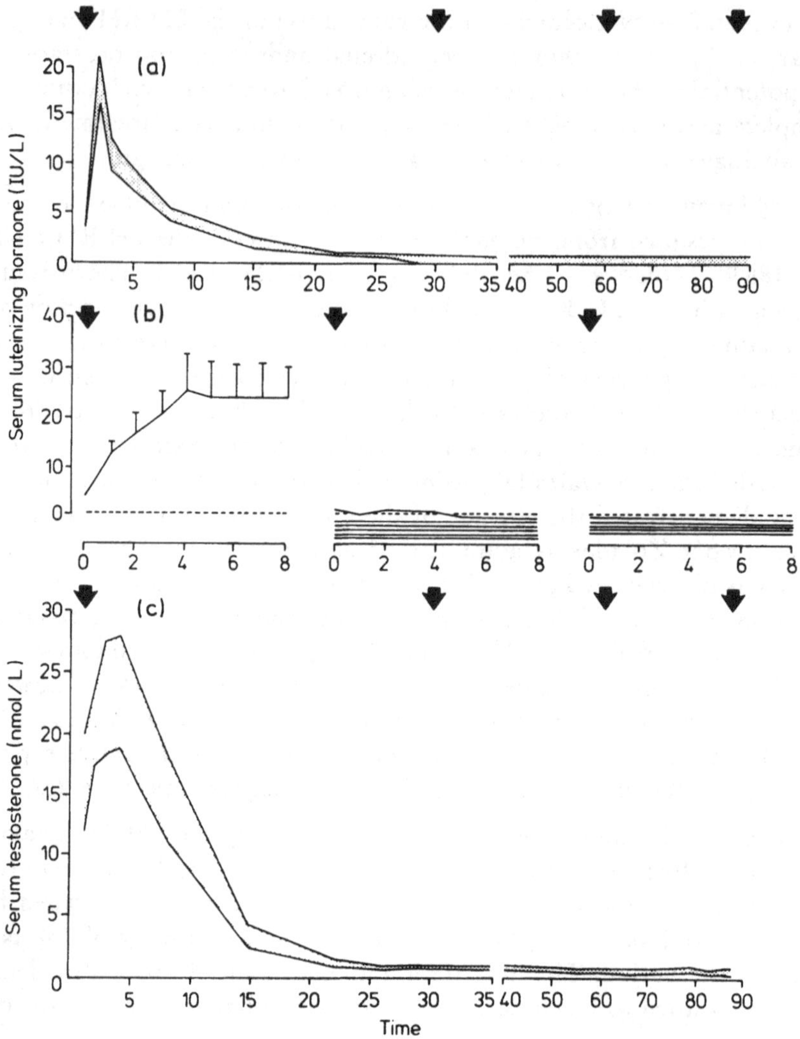

Fig. 3 Changes in the plasma concentrations of luteinizing hormone (LH) and testosterone in patients with prostatic cancer following long term treatment with Zoladex (3.6 mg depot preparation administered every 4 weeks). Arrows indicate when Zoladex was administered and the shaded areas represent the range of values (mean ± s. e. m.). The time is shown in days in Figs. 3 a and 3 c, and as hours in 3 b. Bars in Fig. 3 b indicate ± s. e. m.

or very quickly relapse after a brief response. Research should continue to attempt to identify those 'high risk' patients soon after presentation so that more effective therapy may be considered. Results from Cox Proportional Hazard analysis of data from patients studied by the Tenovus Institute on behalf of the British Prostate Study Group [59] suggest that a 'prognostic index' may be derived from plasma concentrations of testosterone and growth hormone, which together with histological assessment of tumour grade, could offer a rational means of patient selection for primary cytotoxic therapy. A similar approach by Adlercreutz and his colleagues [42] directs attention to plasma testosterone/oestradiol-17β ratios to determine the patients who may respond to endocrine therapy. Certainly with the potential of androgen receptor analysis for such patient selection still to be established [19], this approach may well offer an interesting basis on which to develop new clinical studies.

Summary

The basis of treatment for advanced prostate cancer, first established by Huggins in early 1940's, is the removal of testosterone on which normal and carcinomatous prostate depends for its growth and maintenance. Orchidectomy and diethylstilboestrol (DES), the synthetic oestrogen, have therefore been the main features of treatment for four decades. The cardiovascular problems caused by the use of DES and the concern that only 70% of the patients initially responded to this form of therapy and in most, the disease recurred shortly, caused widespread search for new treatment methods to continue. Various progestational steroids have been used for primary therapy but their effectiveness are yet to be established by randomised trials. Efforts have also been made to further decrease the small amounts of circulating androgens of adrenal origin following or in combination with primary endocrine therapy. Recently luteinizing hormone-releasing hormone analogues (LH-RH) have become the centre of worldwide interest in the treatment of prostate cancer. Early investigations indicated that Zoladex, a depot LH-RH analogue administered every 28 days, produced medical castration and a Phase III randomised trial was established in the U. K. to study the clinical potential of this drug against orchidectomy. Interim reports on the trial incorporating 358 patients with advanced disease suggests that objective and subjective rates of response during the first 15-months follow-up period and the preliminary survival figures are similar in both groups. The drug is well-tolerated with minimal side effects. This study therefore clearly indicates that Zoladex provides a valuable alternative for the treatment of prostate cancer.

References

[1] Abramson, F. P., H. C. Miller Jr.: Biovailability, distribution and pharmacokinetics of diethylstilboestrol produced from Stilboestrol. J. Urol. **128** (1982) 1336–1339.

[2] Arduino, L. J.: Veterans Administration Cooperative Urological Research Group. Carcinoma of the prostate. Treatment and comparisons. J. Urol. **98** (1967) 516–522.

[3] Bard, D. R., I. Lasnitzki: The influence of oestradiol on the metabolism of androgens by human prostatic tissue. J. Endocrinol. **74** (1977) 1–9.
[4] Bhanalaph, T., M. J. Varkarakis, G. P. Murphy: Current status of bilateral adrenalectomy for advanced prostatic carcinoma. Ann. Surg. **179** (1974) 17–21.
[5] Brendler, H.: Adrenalectomy and hypophysectomy for prostatic cancer. Urology **2** (1973) 99–102.
[6] Burge, P. D., M. E. Harper, M. Hartog et al.: Subcapsular orchidectomy – An effective operation? Proc. Roy. Soc.Med. **69** (1976) 663–664.
[7] Byar, D. P.: VACURG studies on prostatic cancer and its treatment. In: M. Tannenbaum (ed.): Urological pathology: The Prostate, pp. 241–267. Lea and Febiger, New York 1977.
[8] Cowley, T. H., B. G. Brownsey, M. E. Harper, et al.: The effect of ACTH on plasma testosterone and androstenedione concentrations in patients with prostatic carcinoma. Acta Endocrinol. Copenh. **81** (1976) 310–320.
[9] Danutra, V., M. E. Harper, A. R. Boyns et al.: The effect of certain stilboestrol analogues on plasma prolactin and testosterone in the rat. J. Endocrinol. **57** (1973) 207–215.
[10] Drago, J. R., R. J. Santen, A. Lipton et al.: Clinical effects of aminoglutethimide, medical adrenalectomy, in treatment of 43 patients with advanced prostatic carcinoma. Cancer **53** (1984) 1447–1450.
[11] Edsmyr, F., L. Anderson, I. Konyves: Estramustine phosphate (Estracyt); Experimental studies and clinical experience. In: G. H. Jacobi, R. Hohenfeller (eds.): Prostate Cancer, International Perspectives in Urology Vol. 3, pp. 253–266. Williams & Wilkins, Baltimore–London 1982.
[12] Farnsworth, W. E.: the direct effect of estrogens. Invest. Urol. **6** (1969) 423–427.
[13] Fitzpatrick, J. M., R. A. Gardiner, J. P. Williams et al.: Pituitary ablation in the relief of pain in advanced prostatic carcinoma. Br. J. Urol. **52** (1980) 301–304.
[14] Geller, J., G. Vazakas, B. Fruchtman et al.: The effect of cyproterone acetate on adenocarcinoma of the prostate. Surg. Gyn. Ob. **1227** (1968) 748–758.
[15] Geller, J., J. Albert, S. S. C. Yen: Treatment of advanced cancer of the prostate gland with megestrol acetate. Urology **12** (1978) 537–541.
[16] Goodwin, D. A., D. S. Rasmussen-Taxdal, A. O. Ferreira et al.: Estrogen inhibition of androgen-maintained prostatic secretion in the hypophysectomised dog. J. Urol. **86** (1961) 134–136.
[17] Griffiths, K., P. Davies, M. E. Harper et al.: The etiology and endocrinology of prostatic cancer. In: D. Rose (ed.): Endocrinology of Cancer, Vol. 2. pp. 1–55. CRC Press, Florida/Cleveland, Ohio 1979.
[18] Griffiths, K., P. Davies, M. E. Harper et al.: Biochemical effects of cytotoxic estrogens and cytotoxic antioestrogens. In: J. Raus, M. Martens, G. Leclercq (eds.): Cytotoxic Estrogens in Hormone Receptive Tumors, pp. 183–205. Academic Press, 1980.
[19] Griffiths, K., P. Davies, C. L. Eaton et al.: Cancer of the Prostate: Endocrine factors. Oxford Rev. Reprod. Biol. **9** (1987) 192–259.
[20] Harper, M. E., W. B. Peeling, K. Griffiths: Adrenal androgens and the prostate. In: The Proceedings of the International Symposium of Hormone Therapy of Prostatic Disease – Basic and Clinical Aspects, Medicom Europe Apeldoorn (In press) 1988.
[21] Huggins, C., P. J. Clark: Quantitative studies of prostatic secretion. II. The effect of castration and of estrogen injection on the normal and on the hyperplastic prostatic glands of dogs. J. Exp. Med. **72** (1940) 747–762.
[22] Huggins, C., C. V. Hodges: Studies on prostatic cancer. The effect of castration, of estrogen and of androgen injection on serum phosphatases in metastatic carcinoma of the prostate. Cancer Res. **1** (1941) 293–297.
[23] Huggins, C., R. E. Stevens Jr., C. V. Hodges: Studies on prostatic cancer. II. The effects of castration on advanced carcinoma of the prostate gland. Arch. Surg. **43** (1941) 209–223.
[24] Jonsson, G., B. Hogberg: Treatment of advanced prostatic carcinoma with Estracyt: A preliminary report. Scand. J. Urol. Nephrol. **5** (1971) 103–107.
[25] Jonsson, G., A. M. Olsson, W. Luttrop et al.: Treatment of prostatic carcinoma with various types of oestrogen derivatives. In: P. L. Munson, E. Diczfalusy, J. Glover, et al. (eds.): Vitamins and Hormones Vol. 33, pp. 351–376. Academic Press, London 1975.
[26] Jonsson, G., B. Hogberg, T. Nilsson: Treatment of advanced prostatic carcinoma with estramustine phosphate (Estracyt). Scand. J. Urol. Nephrol. **11** (1977) 231–238.

[27] Jordan, W. B.: Jr., C. E. Blackard, D. P. Byar: Reconsideration of orchiectomy in the treatment of advanced prostatic carcinoma. Southern Med. J. **70** (1977) 1411 – 1413.

[28] Kemp, H. A., G. F. Read, D. R. Fahmy et al.: Measurement of diethylstilboestrol in plasma from patients with cancer of the prostate. Cancer Res. **41** (1981) 4693 – 4697.

[29] Labrie, F., A. Dupont, A. Belanger et al.: New approach in the treatment of prostatic cancer. Complete instead of partial withdrawal of androgens. The Prostate **4** (1983) 579 – 594.

[30] Labrie, F., A. Dupont, A. Belanger: Complete androgen blockade for the treatment of prostate cancer. In: V. T. de Vita, S. Hellman, S. A. Rosenberg (eds.): Important advances in oncology, pp. 193 – 217. Lippincott Co., Philadelphia 1985.

[31] Leistenschneider, W., R. Nagel: Estracyt therapy of advanced prostatic cancer with special reference to control of therapy with cytology and DNA-cytophotometry. Eur. Urol. **6** (1980) 111 – 117.

[32] Lukkarinen, O., G. L. Hammond, M. Kontturi et al.: Testicular steroid secretion and peripheral serum steroid concentrations in patients with prostatic carcinoma after short-term oestrogen treatment. Invest. urol. **16** (1979) 453 – 456.

[33] Maynard, P. V., R. I. Nicholson: Effects of high dose of a series of new luteinizing hormone-releasing hormone analogues in intact female rats. Brit. J. Cancer **39** (1979) 274 – 279.

[34] McDonald, J. H., J. A. Calams: Extraparenchymal Leydig-like cells: observations following subcapsular orchidectomy. J. Urol. **82** (1959) 145 – 147.

[35] Mellinger, G. T.: Veterans Administration Cooperative Urological Research Group. Carcinoma of the prostate: a continuing co-operative study. J. Urol. **91** (1964) 500 – 594.

[36] Murray, R., P. Pitt: Treatment of advanced prostatic cancer, resistant to conventional therapy, with aminoglutethimide. Eur. J. Cancer Clin. Oncol. **21** (1985) 453 – 458.

[37] Nesbit, R. M., W. C. Baum: Endocrine control of prostatic carcinoma. J. Amer. med. Ass. **143** (1950) 1317 – 1320.

[38a] Oshima, M., K. Wakabayashi, B. Tamaoki: The effect of synthetic oestrogen upon the biosynthesis in vitro of androgen and luteinizing hormone in the rat. Biochim. Biophys. Acta **137** (1967) 356 – 364.

[38b] Pavone-Macaluso, M., H. de Voogt, G. Viggiano et al.: Comparison of diethylstilbestrol, cyproterone acetate and medroxyprogesterone acetate in the treatment of advanced prostatic cancer: Final analysis of a randomized phase III trial of the european organization for research on treatment of cancer urological group. J. Urol. **136** (1986) 624 – 631.

[39] Peeling, W. B., K. Griffiths: Endocrine treatment of prostatic cancer. In: J. P. Blandy, B. Lytton (eds.): The Prostate, pp. 188 – 207. Butterworths, London 1986.

[40] Peeling, W. B., A. C. Buck, K. Griffiths et al.: A Phase III trial comparing ICI 118630 ("Zoladex") with orchidectomy in the management of advanced prostatic cancer. Brit. J. Urol. (In press) (1988).

[41] Pierrepoint, C. G., A. O. Turkes, K. J. Walker et al.: Endocrine factors in the treatment of prostatic cancer. In: EORTC Genitourinary Group Monograph 2, Part A; Therapeutic principles in metastatic prostatic cancer, pp. 51 – 72. Alan R. Liss Inc., New York 1985.

[42] Rannikko, S., A.-L. Kairento, S.-L. Karonen et al.: Hormonal patterns in prostatic cancer 1. Correlation with local extent of tumour, presence of metastases and grade of differentiation. Acta Endocr. **98** (1981) 625 – 633.

[43] Resnick, M. I., J. T. Grayhack: Treatment of Stage IV carcinoma of the prostate. Urol. Clin. N. Amer. **2** (1975) 141 – 161.

[44] Riba, L. W.: Subcapsular castration for carcinoma of the prostate. J. Urol. **48** (1942) 384 – 387.

[45] Shearer, R. J., W. F. Hendry, I. F. Sommerville et al.: Plasma testosterone. An accurate monitor of hormone treatment in prostatic cancer. Brit. J. Urol. **45** (1973) 668 – 677.

[46] Shimazaki, J., H. Kinhara, I. Yoshikazu et al.: Testosterone metabolism in the prostate; formation of androstan-17beta-ol-3-one and androst-4-ene-3,17-dione and inhibitory effects of natural and synthetic estogens. Gunma. J. Med. Sci. **14** (1965) 313 – 325.

[47] Smith, R. B., P. C. Walsh, W. E. Goodwin: Cyproterone acetate in the treatment of advanced carcinoma of the prostate. J. Urol. **110** (1973) 106 – 108.

[48] Sogani, P. C., W. F. Whitmore: Experience with Flutamide in previously untreated patients with advanced carcinoma of the prostate. J. Urol. (1979) 640 – 643.

[49] Stoliar, B., D. J. Albert: SCH 13521 in the treatment of advanced cancer of the prostate with megestrol acetate. J. Urol. (1974) 803 – 807.
[50] Stone, A. R., T. B. Hargreave, G. D. Chisholm: The diagnosis of oestrogen escape and the role of secondary orchidectomy in prostatic cancer. Br. J. Urol. 52 (1980) 535 – 538.
[51] Susan, L. P., R. B. Roth, W. C. Adkins: Regression of prostatic cancer metastases by high doses of diethylstilboestrol diphospate. Urology 13 (1976) 429 – 434.
[52] Turkes, A. O., W. B. Peeling, K. Griffiths: Treatment of patients with advanced cancer of the prostate: Phase III trial, Zoladex against castration; A study of the British Prostate Group. J. Steroid Biochem. 27 (1987) 543 – 549.
[53] Turkes, A. O., W. B. Peeling, K. Griffiths: Zoladex in the treatment of metastatic prostate cancer. In: Hormones and Cancer, Proceedings of the 3rd International Congress on Hormones and Cancer, Raven Press New York 1987 (In press).
[54] Vermeulen, A., W. Schalfhout, W. De Sy: Plasma androgen levels after capsular orchiectomy or estrogen treatment for prostatic carcinoma. The Prostate 3 (1982) 115 – 121.
[55a] Veronesi, A., F. Zattoni, S. Frustaci et al.: Estramustine phosphate (Estracyt) treatment of T3 – T4 prostatic carcinoma. The Prostate 3 (1982) 159 – 164.
[55b] Voogt, de, H. J., P. H. Smith, M. Pavone-Macaluso et al.: Cardiovascular side effects of diethylstilbestrol, cyproterone acetate, medroxyprogesterone acetate and estramustine phosphate used for the treatment of advanced prostatic cancer: Results from european organization for research on treatment of cancer trials 30761 and 30762. J. Urol. 135 (1986) 303 – 307.
[56] Walker, K. J., R. I. Nicholson, A. O. Turkes et al.: Therapeutic potential of the LHRH agonist, ICI 118630, in the treatment of advanced prostatic carcinoma. Lancet, August (1983), 413 – 415.
[57] Walker, K. J., A. O. Turkes, A. Turkes: Treatment of patients with advanced cancer of the prostate using a slow-release (depot) formulation of the LHRH agonist ICI 118630 (Zoladex (R)). J. Endocr. 103 (1984) R1 – R4.
[58] Whitmore, W. F.: The natural history of prostatic cancer. Cancer 32 (1973) 1104 – 1112.
[59] Wilson, D. W., M. E. Harper, H. M. Jensen et al.: A prognostic index for the clinical management of patients with advanced prostatic cancer: A British Prostate Study Group investigation. Prostate 7 (1985) 131 – 141.

Rationale of total androgen blockade by cyproterone acetate*

U. W. Tunn

Introduction

The basic principles of total androgen blockade in prostatic cancer must be based on the realisation of two problems. One is the pharmacological problem of androgen deprivation, the other the reaction of the tumor cell after androgen withdrawal. In the previous chapters of this book the endocrinological principles of androgen withdrawal and the reaction of androgen dependent target cells have been dealt with extensively. The problems of the clinical application of androgen withdrawal in prostatic cancer should be discussed. This will lead to the basic limitations of total androgen blockade.

Clinical principles and problems of total androgen blockade

Total or complete androgen deprivation is defined as simultaneous withdrawal of testicular and adrenal androgens. This therapeutic principle has been practised for 10 years in the treatment of prostatic cancer using cyproterone acetate (CPA) as a pharmacological monotherapy [7, 11, 12]. Labrie and coworkers [5] recently pushed the term complete androgen deprivation to new highlights of publicity. They completed androgen withdrawal by combining a LH-RH agonist with a non-steroidal antiandrogen. They assumed that this therapy was superior to all other standard therapies.

It is the intention of complete androgen deprivation to achieve a milieu free of androgens in the prostate. In principle this is possible by monotherapy or combination therapy. Table 1 summarizes the possibilities of elimination of testicular and adrenal androgens. The so-called complete androgen deprivation can be achieved by high doses of CPA as a monotherapy or by a combination

* This article is dedicated to Prof. Dr. Theodor Senge on occasion of his 50th birthday.

New Developments in Biosciences 4

Table 1 Basic possibilities of complete androgen deprivation

1. Antiandrogens with antigonadotropic effect (high-dosed CPA)
2. Surgical Castration Plus Antiandrogen (CPA or flutamide)
3. Medicinal Castration (LH-RH agonist) Plus Antiandrogen (CPA or flutamide)

of surgical or pharmacological castration with steroidal and non-steroidal antiandrogens.

Neumann dealt in this book with the differences of steroidal and non-steroidal antiandrogens. It is to be underlined in this context that CPA can be given in high doses as a monotherapy because of its additional antigonadotropic effect.

Antiandrogens of the non-steroidal type like flutamide and anandrone neutralize androgen stimulation of the target organ like CPA. They also compete with androgens for receptors in neural centers. The result is an increased gonadotropin secretion resulting in increased testosterone biosynthesis. So pure antiandrogens induce a rise of serum testosterone concentration in the patient with his testes intact and increase the intracellular bioavailability of dihydrotestosterone (DHT) in the prostate. CPA reduces the intraprostatic DHT bioavailability. Its pharmacological characteristic makes it an example for achieving total androgen deprivation.

The problem of prostatic cancer is not only total androgen deprivation but also androgen sensitivity of the tumor cells [4]. Prostatic cancer could be treated curatively by androgen deprivation if all tumor cells were androgen sensitive. Clinical experience tells otherwise. Prostatic cancer can be controlled by androgen withdrawal only for a limited amount of time. Despite a so called total androgen deprivation tumor progression is possible for two reasons:

1. Heterogeneity of tumor cells with androgen sensitive and androgen insensitive cells
2. Insufficient androgen blockade on the cellular level.

Tumor cell heterogeneity: morphological, immunohistochemical and biochemical examples

First some remarks regarding heterogeneity of tumor cells.

Experimental investigations by Isaacs [3, 4] have defined the responses to androgen withdrawal in three populations of prostatic cancer cells:

1. Androgen-dependent cells: These cells require continuous androgen supply for their existence and die after androgen withdrawal.
2. Androgen sensitive tumor cells: These cancer cells survive without androgens, but have a higher growth rate in the presence of androgens.
3. Androgen independent tumor cells: The growth of these tumor cells is not at all influenced by androgens.

Transferring this model to the clinical setting the initial response of the individual heterogeneous prostatic cancer to androgen deprivation is defind by the pre-existing relation of androgen dependent, androgen sensitive and androgen insensitive tumor cells. Androgen withdrawal controls the androgen sensitive tumor part only. Androgen resistance of the individual prostatic cancer which is based on tumor cell heterogeneity can be demonstrated in human prostatic cancer morphologically, biochemically and enzymhistochemically. In cooperation with G. Aumüller, Universität Marburg, Anatomisches Institut, we have done some investigations on tissue specimens of radical prostatectomy in patients who had been treated with CPA preoperatively in a dosage of 300 mg per week for 2 months.

Morphologically we found marked regressive changes of the prostatic carcinoma after the short-term adjuvant CPA-therapy. Therapy – induced regression shows especially in the disseminated and reduced numbers of tumor cells and in the vacuolisation of carcinoma cells with nuclear pycnosis and fibrosed stroma. In one prostatectomy specimens we find regression patterns of various tumor cells with low and high grade regression.

Furthermore, the unlabelled antibody enzyme method was used for the detection of prostatic phosphatase in the prostatectomy specimens. After pre-operative CPA treatment we found in all prostatectomy specimens significantly reduced immunohistochemical evidence of phosphatases. Residual activities could be demonstrated in all sections examined so far. The distribution pattern was irregular as in figure 1, where numerous immuno-reactive tumor cells can be found together with non-reactive cells.

The different biochemical character of prostatic cancer cells is for example apparent in their 5-alpha-reductase activity. Together with H. U. Schweikert, Med. Universitäts-Poliklinik Bonn, we have measured enzym activities in biopsies of prostatic cancer according to Schweikert's [10] method comparing it to BPH tissue.

Schweikert's method allows to analyse testosterone metabolism and morphology in the same tissue sample. We investigated 118 tissue samples of 23 patients. Figure 2 shows the DHT production rate (pmo 1 $\times$ 100 mg^{-1} $\times$ 30 min.$^{-1}$) of BPH and untreated prostatic cancer. There is no difference between BPH and G I prostatic cancer tissue. There is a significant difference between G II and G III

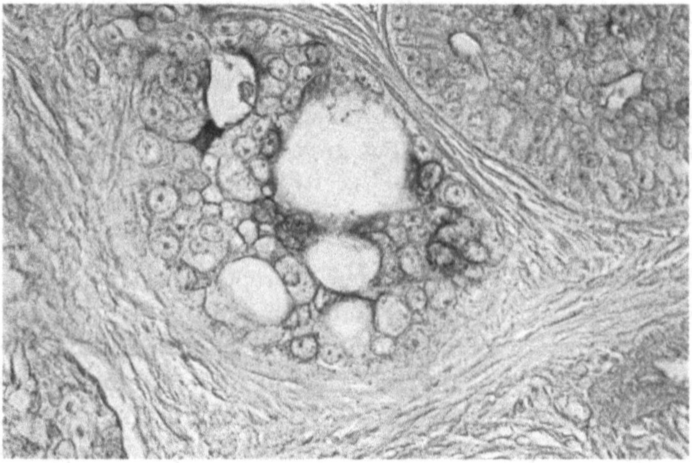

a

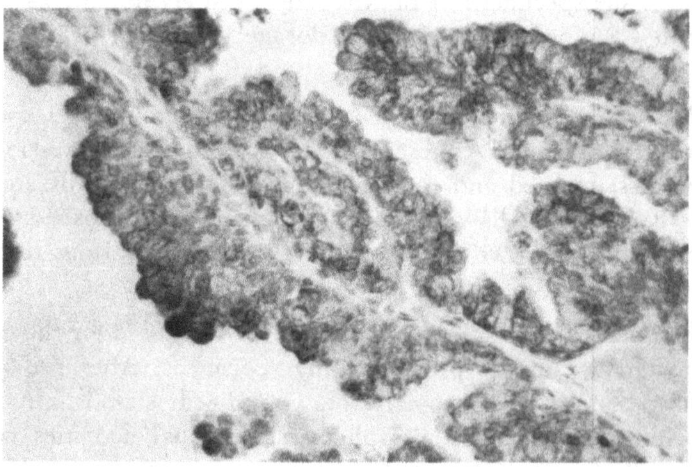

b

Fig. 1 Immunohistochemical demonstration of acid phosphatase (AP):
1a Normal prostate: the reaction product is localized at the apical portion of the columnar cells.
1b Prostatic carcinoma after 6-weeks CPA-treatment: AP immunreactivity is absent in most carcinoma cells.

prostatic cancer tissue with a reduction factor of 6.5. Furthermore, we analysed the testosterone metabolism in tissue samples of patients who had been treated with complete androgen deprivation by castration and CPA for at least 1 year and who were clearly in remission or progression at that time. With this experimental setting we wanted to find out whether testosterone metabolism is different in patients with differing prognosis.

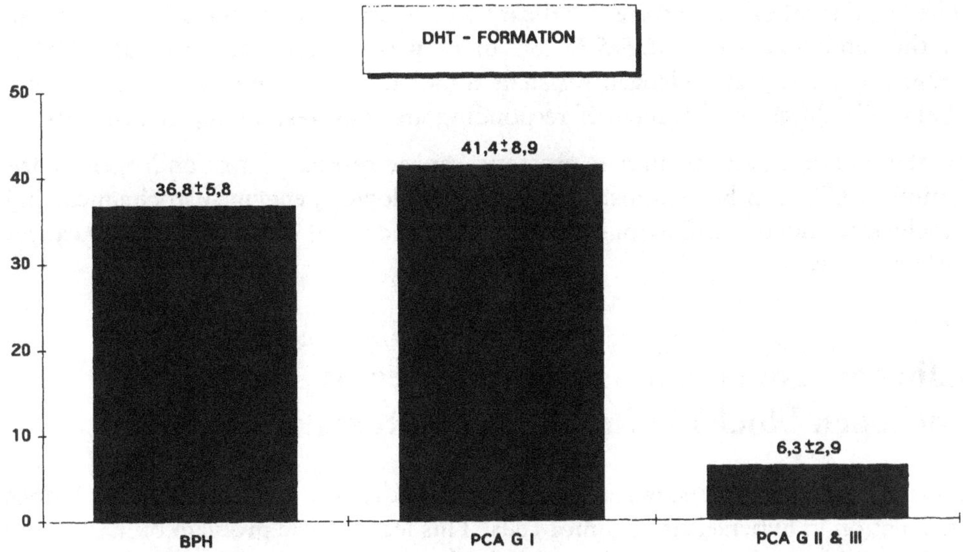

a

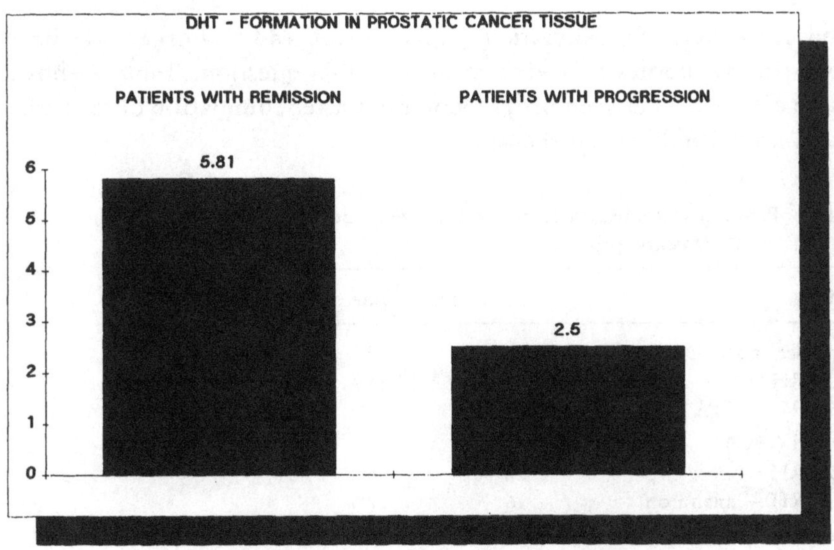

b

Fig. 2 DHT production rate (pmol × 100 mg^{-1} × 30 min^{-1}) of prostatic tissue:

2a Benign prostatic hyperplasia (BPH), Grade I – prostatic carcinom (CPA G I), grade G II & grade G III – prostatic carcinoma (PCA G II & G III).

2b G II & G III prostatic cancer tissue from patientes with remission and progression treated with CPA for at least 1 year.

The DHT synthesis rate were significantly different in the progression group and in the remission group (2.5/5.8). So there was a significant loss of 5-alpha-reductase activity in androgen resistent tumor cells. This demonstrates the biochemically different character of responding and non-responding tumor cells.

So the heterogeneity of human prostatic cancer response after androgen deprivation by CPA can be demonstrated by morphological, enzymehistochemical and biochemical methods. Obviously androgen withdrawal controls prostatic cancer only partially.

Clinical results comparing total versus subtotal androgen blockade in advanced prostatic cancer

Labrie [5] stated that smallest amounts of androgens are sufficient to induce stimulation in hypersensitive tumor cells. This leads to the problem of inadequate androgen blockade on the cellular level. If only complete androgen deprivation leads to adequate androgen withdrawal progression rates in prostatic cancer should be higher after elemination of testicular androgens only than after combination therapy.

Schröder and coworkers [9], Navratil [6] and Brisset and coworkers [1] have published prospective studies this year to answer this question. Table 2 shows that there is no difference between progression rates after elimination of testicular androgens and after combination therapy.

Table 2 Prospective studies on complete androgen blockade in patients with metastatic prostate cancer

authors	no. of pts.	rate of progression
Schroeder et al. (1987)		
– LH-RH	58	38%
– LH-RH + CPA	13	41%
Navratil (1987)		
– LH-RH	22	45%
– LH-RH + anandron	16	37%
Brisset et al. (1987)		
– castration	43	42%
– castration + anandron	46	43%

In an earlier prospective randomised study we had compared the therapeutic effectivity of CPA monotherapy with a standard estrogen therapy [12]. There were no significant differences in 5 years survival. It was 24% in the estrogen group, 26% in the CPA group. Regarding only the M_0-patients we found a 5 years survival of 52% in the CPA group and 43% in the estrogen group. Statistical analysis showed no significant differences. Considering these results you have to remember that the CPA dose of 100 mg per day has to be regarded as to small today. We demand a dose of 300 mg i.m. per week or 200 mg per os per day in CPA monotherapy today.

So far there is no biochemical evidence of complete androgen deprivation in human prostatic tissue. We have investigations done by Voigt and Bartsch [13] and by Geller and coworkers [2]. They examined DHT concentrations in prostatic cells and selectively in the nucleus. After 6 weeks of treatment with 300 mg CPA i.m. per week Voigt found high CPA concentrations in serum and prostatic tissue but only incomplete DHT reduction in the nucleus. Geller and coworkers examined DHT tissue concentrations of BPH patients with transurethral resection after 14 days of flutamide treatment.

They found a 40% reduction of DHT in the cytosol, but no significant difference in the nuclear fraction. The question whether in vivo complete androgen deprivation can really achieve a milieu 100% free of androgens in the prostate has to be considered again in the light of these investigations. These findings justify the therapeutic concept of the so-called complete androgen blockade and of not taking the slightest therapeutic risk. It has to be mentioned in this context that we have no reliable information on which amount of androgen in vivo can stimulate a prostatic tumor cell.

Behaviour of the primary tumor and of metastases

The question arises whether primary tumor and metastases are influenced simultaneously by androgen deprivation. In 72 patients with metastasising prostatic cancer we have compared the behaviour of prostatic volume with that of the metastases. The clinical result after 1 year of antiandrogenic therapy was graded according to the evaluation criteria of the EORTC [8] complete remission, partial remission, no change and progression which describes the behaviour of metastases especially. Prostatic volumes were examined before therapy and after 12 months by transrectal sonography. This shows us the reaction of the primary tumor to androgen deprivation. In the few patients with complete remission there was a significant reduction of prostatic volume of 84%. The reduction of prostatic volume in the partial remission and no change groups was less, and there was no significant difference between these groups. In the progression group we found an amount reduction of 37%.

So as a tendency we find a correlation between the behaviour of the primary tumor and of the metastases. Especially there is a significant difference in volume reduction between patients with complete remission and progression, although in progression we also find a volume reduction of 37%. Prostatic volume reduction is not significantly different in patients whose reaction in the metastases is defined as partial remission or no change. Like in the primary tumor the behaviour of metastases after androgen deprivation depends on the ratio of androgen dependent and independent prostatic cancer cell phenotypes.

Concluding remarks

In summary the conclusion is that all kinds of androgen deprivation including complete androgen withdrawal with CPA in advanced prostatic cancer are palliative measures. The primarily heterogeneous composition of prostatic cancer makes curative treatment impossible. Androgen withdrawal influences only the androgen dependent part of the tumor. Androgen deprivation should block all androgenic stimulations on the cellular level with therapeutic security and few side effects.

In the clinic the potent antiandrogen CPA can be used for androgen blockade as a monotherapy in a high dose or in a low dose in combination with surgical or pharmacological castration so that the tumor cells which can be stimulated by androgens are blocked. So the problem is solved how to control androgen dependent tumor parts. In the future our attention should center on finding effective therapy principles against those parts of the tumor which are androgen insensitive and hardly controllable. The patient's fate will be determined by the androgen independent tumor part ultimately.

References

[1] Brisset, J. M., L. Boccon-Gibod, H. Botto et al.: Anandron (RU 23908) associated to surgical castration in previously untreated stage D prostate cancer: A multicenter comparative Study of two doses of the drug an of a placebo. In: Murphy, G. P., S. Khoury, R. Küss et al. (eds.): Prostate Cancer, pp. 411–422, Alan R. Liss, Inc., New York 1987.

[2] Geller, J., J. Albert, D. A. Nachtheim et al.: The effects of flutamide on total DHT and nuclear DHT levels in the human prostate. Prostate 2 (1981) 309–314.

[3] Isaacs, J. T.: The timing of androgen ablation therapy and/or chemotherapy in the treatment of prostatic cancer. The prostate 5 (1984) 1–18.

[4] Isaacs, J. T.: New principles in the management of metastatic prostatic cancer. Prog. Clin. Biol. Res. **185A** (1985) 303–405.

[5] Labrie, F., A. Dupont, A. Belanger et al.: New hormonal therapy in prostatic carcinoma: combined treatment with an LHRH agonist and an antiandrogen. Clin. Invest. Med. 5 (1982) 267–275.

[6] Navratil, H.: Double-blind study of anandron versus placebo in stage D_2 prostate cancer patients receiving buserelin. In: G. P. Murphy, S. Khoury, R. Küss et al. (eds.): Prostate Cancer, pp. 401–410, Alan R. Liss, Inc., New York 1987.

[7] Neumann, F.: Experimental basis for the clinical use of antiandrogens. In: N. Bruchovsky, A. Chapdelaine, F. Neumann (eds): Regulation of androgen action, pp. 43 – 49, R. Brückner, Berlin 1985.

[8] Schroeder, F. H. and the European Organization for Research on Treatment of Cancer Urological Group: Treatment response criteria for prostatic cancer. Prostate 5 (1984) 181 – 191.

[9] Schroeder, F. H., T. Lock, D. R. Chada et al.: Metastatic cancer of the prostate managed with buserelin versus buserelin plus cyproterone acetate. J. Urol. 137 (1987) 912 – 918.

[10] Schweikert, H. U., P. J. Funke, U. W. Tunn: Androgene und Prostatakarzinom: Testosteronmetabolismus im menschlichen Prostatakarzinom. In: B. Helpap, Th. Senge, W. Vahlensiek (eds): Prostatakarzinom, pp. 12 – 18, pmi-Verlag, Frankfurt – Zürich 1984.

[11] Tunn, U. W., J. Graff, Th. Senge: Treatment of inoperable prostatic cancer with cyproterone acetate. In: F. H. Schroeder (ed.): Androgens and Anti-androgens, pp. 149 – 159, Schering Nederland-Weesp 1983.

[12] Tunn, U. W.: Antiandrogene in der Therape des fortgeschrittenen Prostatakarzinoms. In: R. Nagel (ed.): Konservative Therapie des Prostatakarzinoms, pp. 113 – 121, Springer-Verlag, Berlin, Heidelberg, New York 1987.

[13] Voigt, K. P., W. Bartsch: Intratissular androgens in benign prostatic hyperplasia and prostatic cancer. J. steroid Biochem. 25 (1986) 749 – 757.

Clinical experience with Androcur® in the treatment of prostatic cancer

H. Becker, H. Klosterhalfen

The standard treatment of advanced prostate cancer is since 1941 bilateral orchiectomy or estrogen application [4]. Because of the severe side effects of estrogens orchiectomy is the favoured treatment by many urologists. Testosterone in plasma is reduced rapidly after orchiectomy, already 24 hours after the operation the testosterone values were found to be in the castration level [9], compared to the modern treatment with LH-RH analogues this may be an advantage.

Table 1 Serum testosterone concentrations (μg/l) before and after orchiectomy

	Before treatment	After orchiectomy
Young + Kent	5.6	0.5
Robinson + Thomas	6.07	0.3
Mackler et al.	6.2	0.5
Shearer et al.	2.8	0.47
Bartsch et al.	4.4	0.23

Testosterone in plasma after orchiectomy was found in a range between 0.2 – 0.5 μg/l (table 1). The residual androgens (about 10% of the total androgens before orchiectomy) are mostly produced in the adrenal cortex. It is unclear how much of the androgens originating from the adrenal cortex are metabolised to androstendione and testosterone and influence on this way the growth of prostate tumors.

In 1968 Klosterhalfen started a prospective randomised study in advanced prostate cancer in which after orchiectomy the residual androgens were inactivated or further lowered by several additional endocrine manipulation (table 2):

Table 2 Endocrine treatment of advanced prostatic carcinoma

1. Basic therapy:	Bilateral orchiectomy
2. Additionally endocrine treatment – randomized:	
.1 Diethylstilbendiphosphate	3 × 120 mg/day
.2 Prednisone	2 × 5 mg/day
.3 Cyproterone acetate	2 × 50 mg/day
.4 Placebo	

New Developments in Biosciences 4

The rationale of this different endocrine principles was in group 1, that in the studies of Nesbit and Baum [6] the best 5 year survival data in stage C were seen with the combination of orchiectomy and estrogens, additionally an effect was expected by the increase of SHBG (sex hormone binding globuline) after diethylstilbendiphosphate, which might bind androgens and a direct cytotoxic effect of diethylstilbendiphosphate was discussed in animal models. Prednisone influences the adrenal cortex by reducing the ACTH concentration from the hypophysis, this should result in a reduced stimulation of the adrenal cortex and leed to a reduced output of adrenal androgens. Cyproterone acetate in group 3 was expected to inactivate the residual androgens in the prostate cancer cells. In 1968 cyproterone acetate was the only available antiandrogen. At that time no data were known about the antiandrogen dosis which is necessary to inactivate the androgens. Our patients received 100 mg cyproterone acetate per day. The patients of group 4 were orchiectomised and received no further endrocrine treatment.

In stage C radiation by supervoltage therapy was performed to the prostate with 60 – 70 Gy, whereas patients with metastatic prostate cancer received the endocrine treatmentd only.

Hormones in plasma

Testosterone and prolactin in plasma were measured under this treatment. Testosterone values were reduced significantly from 4.37 µg/l to 0.18 µg/l 1 week after orchiectomy and 0.23 µg/l after 6 weeks. The prolactin levels were not influenced by orchiectomy (table 3).

Table 3 Hormones in plasma after orchiectomy

	Patients n	Testosterone µg/l	Prolactin µ/l
Before treatment	32	4.37 (7.73 – 5.12)	7.55 (5.85 – 9.75)
1 week after orchiectomy	25	0.18* (0.13 – 0.23)	5.86 (5.02 – 6.85)
6 weeks after orchiectomy	32	0.23* (0.18 – 0.29	6.23 (5.09 – 7.62)

* $p < 0.001$

Table 4 Hormones in plasma after orchiectomy and additional endocrine treatment

	Testosterone			Prolactin		
Additional endrocrine treatment	6 weeks after orchiectomy	1 week after addit. treatment	3 months after addit. treatment	6 weeks after orchiectomy	1 week after addit. treatment	3 months after addit. treatment
Honvan	0.29	0,16		7.52	22.4 $p < 0.001$	
Prednisolone	0.13	0.05 $p < 0.05$	0.08 $p < 0.01$	4.42	4.68	5.02
Baycaron	0.15	0.16	0.28	6.00	6.38	6.88
Androcur	0.29		0.13	6.88	7.26	11.2 $p < 0.02$
Placebo	0.28	0.39	0.18	6.98	8.47	5.86

The testosterone levels showed a further significant reduction only in the treatment group receiving prednisone. No alteration of testosterone could be observed in the other treatment groups. A significant increase of prolactin was seen after cyproterone acetate and after diethylstilbendiphosphate, cyproterone acetate did not leed to prolactin levels above normal values (table 4).

Results of the randomised study

78 patients with metastatic prostate cancer were treated in this randomised study. After 1 year 67% had an incomplete remission, the remission rate was highest in the cyproterone group (77%) and in the prednisone group (73%), whereas in both other groups the remission rate was lower (56%). The remission curves are parallel and showed no significant differences. After 5 years the remission rate in the cyproterone acetate group was 11%, in the diethylstilbendiphosphate group 6%, in the prednisone group 9% and in the placebo group 6%. There was no significance. Only 1 patient out of the cyproterone acetate group with histological proven cancer in the bones showed a tumour remission after 10 years (fig. 1).

Patients with tumour progression received in the diethylstilbendiphosphate, the prednisone and the placebo group cyproterone acetate and after further progression estramustin and after tumor progression in the cyproterone acetate group also estramustin. Further tumour remission after estramustin treatment could be

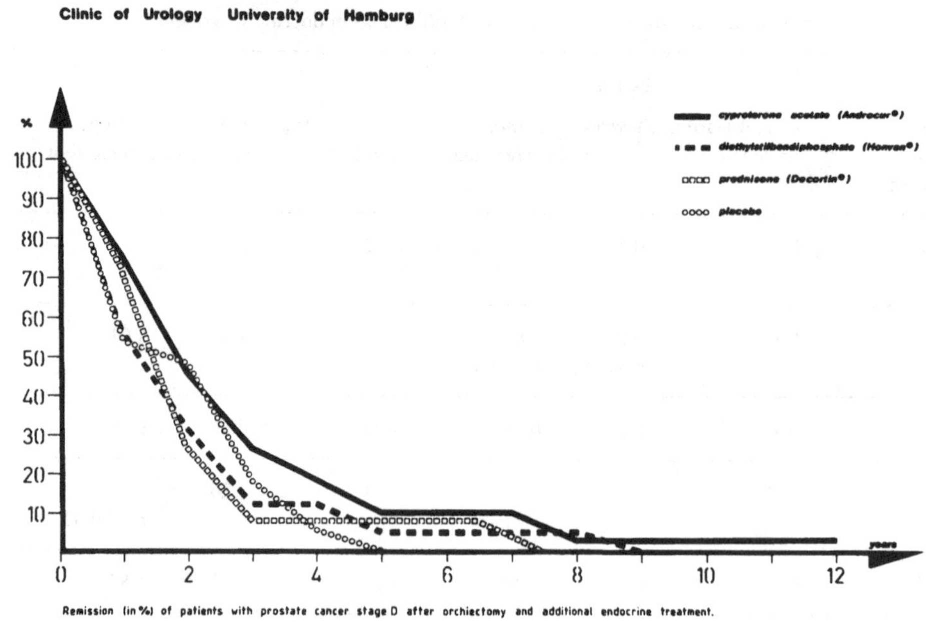

Fig. 1 Remission curves in patients with prostate cancer stage D2 after orchiectomy and additional endocrine treatment.

Table 5 Survival rate in patients with prostate cancer stage D2 after combined endocrine treatment

Additional endrocr. therapy	Patients	1 Year		2 Years		5 Years		10 Years	
	n	n	%	n	%	n	%	n	%
Diethylstilbendiphosphate	24	18	75%	10	42%	2	8%	–	
Prednisone	12	10	83%	7	58%	3	25%	–	
Cyproterone acetate	26	22	85%	16	62%	6	23%	1	4%
Placebo	16	13	81%	11	69%	1	6%	1	6%
Total	78	63	81%	44	56%	12	15%	2	3%

observed very seldom. The survival time after 1 year for all patients was 81% and after 2 years 56%, and after 5 years 15%, i.e. after 5 years only 12 out of 78 patients were alive (table 5). After 5 years survival rate was found in the prednison group (25%) and in the cyproterone acetate group (23%). Statistically there were no significant alterations. Only 2 patients lived longer than 10 years, 1 patient out of the cyproterone acetate group without changing the treatment. The second patient received first of all after orchiectomy no additionally endocrine therapy, after tumour progression he received firstly cyproterone acetate and than a transnasal hypophysectomy was performed. This patient showed after 10 years a tumour progression again and died on his tumour.

Mode of action of antiandrogens at the cellular level

Antiandrogens compete with androgens for the cytoplasmatic androgen receptor. They displace androgens competitively from their receptor binding. We were interested to find out the antiandrogen dosis which is necessary to displace the androgens form the receptor, especially in prostate cancer after orchiectomy. The investigation could only be performed in carcinomatous tissue, and this was not available for us. Therefore we decided to do this studies in patients undergoing prostatectomy in benign prostate hypertrophy [1]. One group of patients received 300 mg cyproterone acetate 3 days before the operation and the second group was treated with 300 mg cyproterone acetate per week 6 weeks before prostatectomy, the last intramuscular injection was given 3 days before the operation. The amounts of cyproterone acetate and testosterone were measured in plasma and of cyproterone acetate and 5α-DHT in bph, whereas in bph the investigations were done in the whole tissue and in the nuclear fraction of stroma and of epithelium. Figure 2 demonstrates the curves of cyproterone acetate values in plasma 3 days after the antiandrogen application compared to 6 weeks regimen. Testosterone in plasma was reduced in both treatment groups, more pronounced in the 6 weeks course (fig. 3). Table 6 demonstrates the reduction of testosterone in plasma and of 5α-DHT in whole tissue and in the nuclear fraction of epithelial

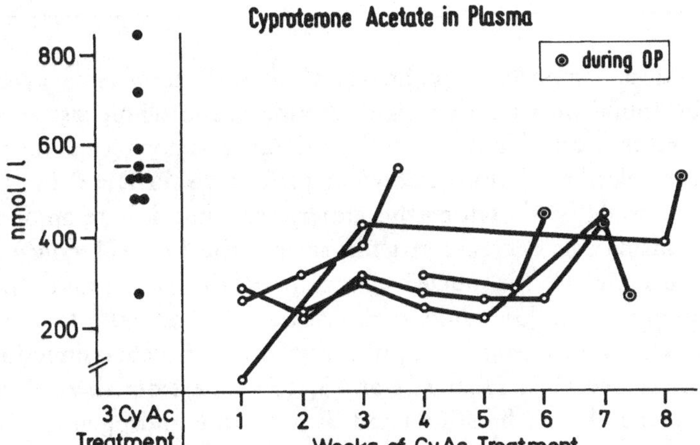

Fig. 2 Cyproterone acetate concentration in plasma.

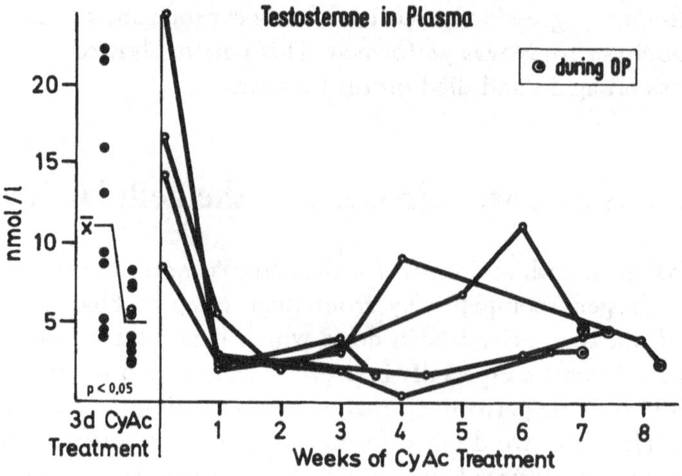

Fig. 3 Plasma testosterone after cyproterone acetate treatment.

Table 6 Testosterone in plasma and 5α-DHT in bph tissue after treatment with cyproterone acetate

	n	Plasma Testosterone (nmol/e)	DHT in Tissue (pmol/mg DNA)		
			WT	SN	EN
Untreated	15	10.9 ± 2.2	7.1 ± 1.1	7.1 ± 0.9	3.8 ± 0.4
3 d CyAc	10	5.0 ± 2.1*	8.5 ± 2.0	6.9 ± 1.1	5.1 ± 1.4
6 w CyAc	4	3.8 ± 1.1*	2.5 ± 0.5*	4.8 ± 1.5	2.3 ± 0.3*

$\bar{x} \pm$ sem; * $p < 0.05$ compared to controls
WT = whole tissue. SN = nuclear fraction of stroma EN = nuclear fraction of epithelium

and stroma fraction compared to controls. Compared to plasma cyproterone acetate could be found in a relative high amount in the whole tissue, whereas only small amounts were found in both nuclear fractions (fig. 4). Figure 5 demonstrates the relation of testosterone in plasma to 5α-DHT in the tissue compartiments. It could be shown by this experiment that despite an decrease of testosterone in plasma this decrease was not seen in the 5α-DHT concentrations in the tissue especially in the nuclear fraction of the epithelium. In animal experiments Huang et al. [3] could demonstrate that an 40-fold increase of cyproterone acetate over androgens did not leed to a complete competion of the androgens from the receptor. Huang et al. [3] conclude from these results that the prostate must be able to be stimulated by very low androgen levels. If this holds true in prostate cancer has to be investigated. Some data show in this direction.

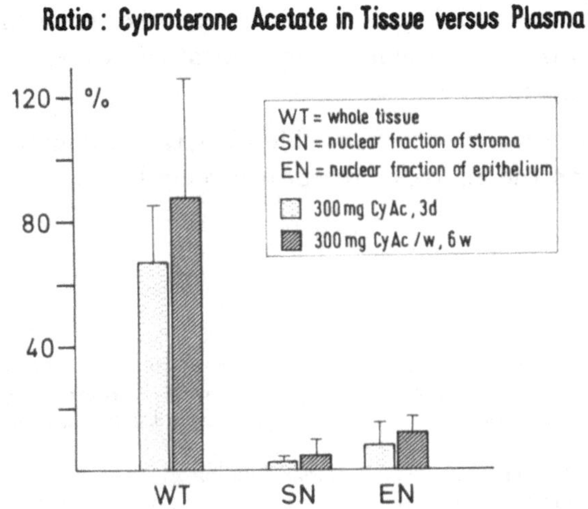

Fig. 4 Cyproterone acetate in bph tissue compared to plasma.

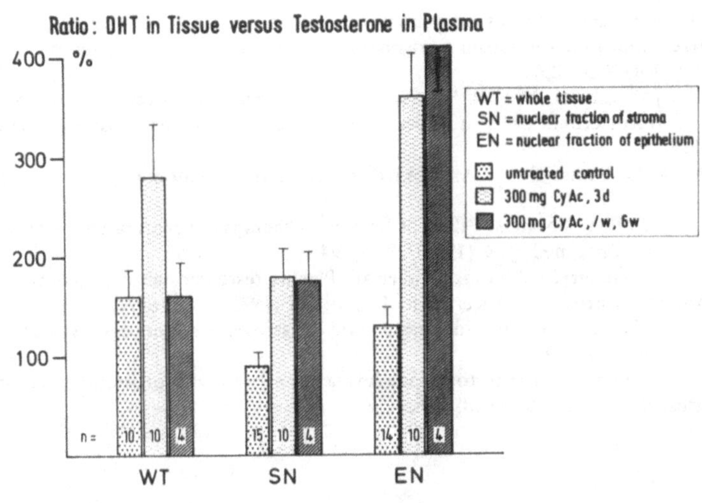

Fig. 5 Ratio: 5α-DHT in tissue versus testosterone in plasma.

Conclusion

1. The residual androgens after orchiectomy may play an important role in prostate cancer growth.
2. An additional antiandrogenic treatment after orchiectomy is favoured in our clinic. More studies are necessary to find out, which antiandrogen shows better results and which dosis of the antiandrogen is necessary to inactivate

the androgens in the tumour cells. The compliance is another problem in the long-term treatment with the old patients – in clinical trials therefore drug monitoring should be performed.

3. From the present data it seems to be impossible to obtain a complete competition of androgens form the androgen receptor protein by antiandrogens.

References

[1] Bartsch, W., H. Becker, B. Düsterberg et al.: 5α-dihydrotestosterone concentration in tissue of benign prostatic hypertrophy following treatment of patients with cyproterone acetate. 4. Congress of the European Society for Urological Oncology and Endocrinology, Amsterdam 1985.

[2] Bartsch, W., H. J. Horst, H. Becker et al.: Sex hormone binding globulin binding capacity, testosterone, 5α-dihydrotestosterone, estradiol and prolactin in plasma of patients with prostatic carcinoma and various types of hormonal treatment. Acta endocr. (Kbh.) **85** (1977) 650–664.

[3] Huang, J. K., W. Bartsch, K.-D. Voigt: Interactions of an anti-androgen (cyproterone acetate) with the androgen receptor system and its biological action in the rat ventral prostate. Acta endocr. (Kbh.) **109** (1985) 569–576.

[4] Huggins, C., C. V. Hodges: Studies on prostatic cancer. I. The effect of castration, of estrogen and of androgen injection on serum phosphatases in metastatic carcinoma of the prostate. Cancer Res. **1** (1941) 293–297.

[5] Mackler, M. A., J. P. Liberti, M. J. V. Smith et al.: The effect of orchiectomy and various doses of stilbestrol on testosterone levels in patients with carcinoma of the prostate. Invest. Urol. **9** (1972) 423–425.

[6] Nesbit, R. M., W. C. Baum: Endocrine control of prostatic carcinoma. J. A. M. A. **143** (1950) 1317–1320.

[7] Robinson, M. R. G., B. S. Thomas: Effect of hormonal therapy on plasma testosterone levels in prostatic carcinoma. Brit. med. J. **4** (1971) 391–394.

[8] Shearer, R. J., W. F. Hendry, F. Sommerville et al.: Plasma testosterone: An accurate monitor of hormone treatment in prostatic cancer. Brit. J. Urol. **45** (1973) 668–677.

[9] Straube, W., J. S. Braun: Zur Orchidektomie und Oestrogentherapie des Prostatacarcinoms. Urologe A **13** (1974) 198–201.

[10] Young, H. H., J. R. Kent: Plasma testosterone levels in patients with prostatic carcinoma before and after treatment. J. Urol. **99** (1968) 788.

Prostate cancer treatment: tolerance of different endocrine regimens

E. Varenhorst

Introduction

The basis of endocrine treatment of cancer of the prostate is the androgen dependency of the tumour. The androgen effect on the carcinoma can be reduced by inhibition of the testicular androgen biosynthesis by means of orchidectomy (OR) or by treatment with oestrogen (OE), a luteinizing hormone releasing hormone analogue (LHRH-A) or an androgen-receptor blocking antiandrogen such as cyproterone acetate (CPA). Owing to their different modes of action, however, different forms of endocrine treatment are tolerated to different degrees. All forms of treatment have undesirable side effects. Even though OR has been used for nearly 50 years, the adverse effects of this operation, that is, postoperative complications and hot flushes, are incompletely investigated. The most serious side effects are the cardiovascular complications associated with oestrogen treatment [3, 8]. It is essential to establish whether OR and the new endocrine regimens are less dangerous in this respect. We therefore started a series of investigations on the changes in cardiovascular risk factors that take place during different endocrine regimens [16 – 22].

The present report summarizes results, and reviews the literature on the tolerance of different forms of endocrine treatment.

Subjects and methods

All patients investigated had cytologically confirmed, advanced carcinoma of the prostate. They were allocated to different endocrine treatments regardless of the stage of the cancer or complicating disease (tab. 1). They were receiving no other endocrine preparations before starting therapy. Metabolic changes known to be indicators of raised risk of congestive heart failure, thromboembolism, and atherosclerosis were investigated in 16 patients treated with OE, 15 treated with the antiandrogenic drug CPA, and 15 who underwent OR [16 – 18, 21, 22].

New Developments in Biosciences 4

Table 1 Treatment and age of 7 groups of patients with prostatic cancer studied with respect to cardiovascular risk factors and complications of endocrine therapy [7, 16 – 22]

Treatment	Patients n	Age, years mean	range
Oestrogens: Ethinyl oestradiol 0.5 – 1.0 mg orally per day + polyoestradiol phostate 80 – 160 mg intramuscularly once monthly	16	69	51 – 81
Subcapsular orchidectormy	15	73	60 – 84
Cyproterone acetate 200 mg orally per day	15	71	58 – 86
LHRH analogue (ICI 118.630) 25 – 125 μg subcutaneously once daily	15	73	59 – 91
LHRH analogue (ICI 118.630) 3.6 mg subcutaneously once per month	30	72	55 – 84
Subcapsular or total orchidectomy	90	72	53 – 85
Subcapsular or total orchidectomy	141	73	52 – 93

Risk factors for atherosclerosis were recorded in 15 patients given LHRH-A subcutaneously once daily [19]; in 30 men receiving LHRH-A in depot form changes in a risk factor for thromboembolism were noted [20]. All variables were studied before and 2 and 8 weeks after the start of treatment.

In 90 patients who underwent OR the incidence, frequency and severity of hot flushes were investigated by questionnaire [7]. Early postoperative complications and duration of hospital stay were noted in 141 patients who underwent OR (84 subcapsular and 57 total). The operation was performed under epidural (n = 23), spinal (n = 72), general (n = 3), or local (n = 43) anaesthesia, in all cases via a scrotal incision. Details are published elsewhere [16 – 22]

Congestive heart failure

Increased plasma volume might tax the circulatory capacity and contribute to cardiac decompensation [16]. The plasma volume was therefore determined by the ^{131}l-albumin method [16].

Thromboembolism

Reduction in antithrombin III (AT III) and a decrease in fibrinolytic activity indicate heightened risk of thromboembolism. The plasma concentration of AT III was measured by a technique using chromogen substrate. The fibrinolytic activity in small vessels and skin capillaries was determined in biopsy specimens by Todd's histochemical method as modified by Risberg [18].

Atherosclerosis

Raised concentrations of low-density lipoprotein (LDL) and/or very-low-density lipoprotein (VLDL) and/or reduced high-density lipoprotein (HDL) are associated with increased risk of atherosclerotic cardiovascular disease. The VLDL, LDL, and HDL fractions in plasma were separated by ultracentrifugation and heparin-$MnCl_2$ precipitation. The cholesterol (C) and triglyceride concentrations in plasma and in lipoprotein fractions were determined enzymatically [21, 22].

Results

Congestive heart failure

The mean plasma volume increased significantly during OE treatment. The plasma volume was unchanged after OR and during treatment with CPA [16]. LHRH-A was not investigated with regard to this factor.

Thromboembolism

In the OE group all patients showed a significant fall in AT III values and fibrinolytic activity during treatment. No mean change in AT III was found after OR or treatment with LHRH-A, and neither was there any change in fibrinolytic activity after OR. During treatment with CPA the mean AT III concentration and the fibrinolytic activity were significantly increased [17–20].

Atherosclerosis

During OE treatment there was a 25% fall in the LDL-C concentration and a 23% mean rise in the mean HDL-C concentration. The changes in HDL-C and LDL-C concentrations were reflected by marked elevations in the HDL-C/C and HDL-C/LDL-C ratios in plasma. CPA treatment caused a mean fall in HDL-C of 25% and a mean fall in LDL-C of 15–10%. The fraction of plasma C carried in HDL showed a mean fall from 19 to 17%. The mean HDL-C/LDL-C ratio was reduced from 0.27 to 0.22. After OR the mean plasma C and VLDL-C concentrations were slightly raised. No mean changes in plasma lipids or lipoproteins were noted during treatment with the LHRH-A [19, 21, 22].

Hot flushes after OR

Of the 90 patients who underwent OR 66 (73%) experienced hot flushes. The number of hot flushes per 24 hours was 1–3 in 29 patients (44%), 4–10 in 31 (47%), and more than 10 in 6 (9%). 33 (50%) were not toubled by the flushes, 15 (23%) were slightly embarrassed, and 18 (27%) were greatly distressed [7].

Postoperative complications

For 141 patients who underwent OR the hospital stay was 2–18 days (mean 4.6). Early postoperative complications occurred in 16, this group remained in hospital for 2–16 days (mean 7.5).

Haemorrhage occurred in 7 and postoperative infection in 9 patients. The overall complication rate was 11.3%. There was no difference in complication rate between subcapsular or total operations or types of anaesthesia.

Discussion

Oestrogens (OE)

During OE therapy almost all patients develop unwanted side effects including feminization, impotence and loss of libido, enlargement of the breasts, and tenderness of the nipples. Occasionally nausea, vomiting or liver failure occur. Most complications appear during the first 6 months [8–10]. However the most serious problem is the increased incidence of cardiovascular complications [3, 8, 9]. Preexisting cardiovascular disease, old age, and overweight aggravate the risk of cardiovascular events [5, 9]. The increased cardiovascular morbidity and mortality were previously thought to be dependent on either very high doses of OE or a previous history of cardiovascular disease [3]. However, a recent controlled study of low dosage OE versus OR disclosed an increased incidence of cardiovascular complications during OE despite the exclusion of patients above 75 years or with a history of cardiovascular disease [9]. In that study 25% of OE treated patients developed major cardiovascular complications during the first year [9]. The explanation for the increased risk of cardiovascular side effects could be metabolic changes induced by the treatment. In the present study there was a fall in AT III and a decrease in vascular tissue fibrinolytic activity, indicating increased risk of thromboembolism. Other studies have shown an increase in factor VII and fibrinogen and increased platelet aggregability [9], further underlining the heightened risk of thrombosis during OE treatment. The raised plasma volume demonstrated in the present study might lead to congestive heart failure in elderly men. Recent findings of increased basal renin-angiotensin-aldosterone activity during OE treatment suggest an important mechanism behind the increased plasma volume and the raised incidence of congestive heart failure [4].

A possible beneficial effect of the changes in lipids and lipoproteins, i.e. the marked elevation of the HDL/LDL ratio, seems to be of limited or no importance for the short term risk of cardiovascular events in middle aged and elderly men [21].

Orchidectomy (OR)

OR is a simple and rapid surgical procedure that carries no life-threatening complications. Nevertheless it must often be performed in an elderly and unstable patient. In our series of 141 consecutive OR there was a complication rate of about 11% in connection with the operation. The psychological impact of the operation has not been thoroughly investigated. Like other endocrine regiments OR results in loss of libido and potency. Patients who underwent OR showed a significantly lesser tendency to develop mental depression than those treated with OE [2], but OE treated men continued sexual activity with their partner oftener than did orchidectomized patients. Hot flushing is sometimes the most distressing symptom. In our study 73% experienced this, and 27% were greatly distressed. Similar figures have been reported during treatment with LHRH-A [7, 12].

The present studies on cardiovascular risk factors after OR showed no changes in coagulation or the fibrinolytic system and no alteration of the plasma volume. There was only a slight increase in C, mainly VLDL-C, which probably has little effect on the development of atherosclerosis and is of no importance for the short term risk of cardiovascular events in elderly men [22]. In a recent investigation no cardiovascular complications occurred during the year after OR when patients with a past history of cardiovascular disease were excluded [9].

Cyproterone acetate (CPA)

Treatment with CPA in a daily oral dose of 200 – 250 mg or a weekly dose of 300 mg intramuscularly diminished libido and potency to roughly the same extent as did OR and OE [10]; slight enlargement of the breasts was seen in some patients. Temporary restlessness or depression have been reported, as have also hyperglycaemia, fatigue, and fluctuation of body-weight.

In the present studies on cardiovascular risk factors we found raised AT III and increased fibrinolytic activity, contrary changes to those observed during OE treatment [17, 18]. The plasma volume was unchanged [16]. Our findings suggest that CPA treatment carries a lower risk of thromboembolism and congestive heart failure than does treatment with OE. The mean C concentration was lowered because of reduction of HDL and LDL, the HDL/LDL ratio being slightly decreased [21]. The fall in total HDL-C was confirmed in a recent study [11]. However, it seems unlikely that the modest reduction in the HDL/LDL ratio during CPA treatment would influence the risk of cardiovascular complications in elderly men. Clinical experience and randomized phase III studies showed lower incidence of cardiovascular side effects during CPA than during OE treatment [10]. However, a high incidence of cardiovascular complications has been reported in an uncontrolled study [14].

Luteinizing hormone releasing hormone analogues (LHRH-A)

The side effects of LHRH-A are comparable to the complications of OR, with loss of libido and potency apparently in the same range [12]. Breast swelling and tenderness were reported in some cases. Concerning hot flushes, the incidence, the number per day, and the subjective severity were similar to those in patients who underwent OR; roughly three-fourths of patients experienced hot flushes during treatment with LHRH-A [12]. Investigations on the psychological effects suggested at 6 months less fatigue, depression, and anxiety and more cheerfulness and energy during treatment with LHRH-A than after OR, but the differences were not significant [12]. In the present study on cardiovascular risk factors we found no significant changes in AT III concentrations during treatment with an LHRH-A [20]. Like others we found no changes in lipids or lipoproteins [11, 19]. These results tally with clinical experience and results of phase III studies, indicating that LHRH-A should not increase the risk of cardiovascular complications [12].

Because of the initial increase in plasma testosterone that occurs with LHRH-A therapy during the first week of treatment there is a risk of exacerbation of disease-related symptoms. Serious complications have been reported, and transient increase in bone pain during the first week was noted in some patients with skeletal metastases [12]. Nevertheless the potential for disease flare is a concern confined to the few patients with impending neurological involvement or in whom a rapid symptomatic response is imperative.

Summary and clinical implications

The ideal endocrine therapy for advanced carcinoma of the prostate remains to be discovered. All available forms of endocrine treatment have undesirable side effects including loss of libido and potency. Many patients, however, develop no side effects, but we are still unable to foresee individual tolerance before starting treatment. The risk of thromboembolism and congestive heart failure is increased during OE treatment, even in low dosage and even in patients with no previous history of cardiovascular disease. Characteristic side effects of OR are hot flushes and postoperative complications. CPA is associated with a variety of unspecific side effects. A common complication of LHRH-A treatment is hot flushing, and its main disadvantage is the risk of exacerbation of symptoms during the first week of treatment.

The cardiovascular complications of OE treatment in middle aged and elderly men are probably explained by changes in the coagulation-fibrinolytic system and the salt water balance. Because opposite or no changes in these risk factors were observed during OR, CPA and LHRH-A therapy it might be anticipated that such regimens are not associated with altered risk of cardiovascular complications.

However, with regard to CPA and LHRH-A, long-term studies on large clinical series are required before the postulated advantages of these newer forms of endocrine treatment can be established.

The changes in risk factors for cardiovascular complications of different forms of endocrine treatment are summarized in table 2.

Table 2 Summary of effects of orchidectomy and treatment with oestrogens, LHRH analogue, and cyproterone acetate on variables associated with cardiovascular risk in patients with carcinoma of the prostate [16–22]

	Plasma volume	AT III	Fibrinolytic activity	LDL	HDL	HDL/LDL
Orchidectomy	o	o	o	o	o	o
Oestrogens	↑↑	↓↓↓	↓↓	↓↓↓	↑↑↑	↑↑↑
LHRH-analogue	–	o	–	o	o	o
Cyproterone acetate	o	↑	↑	↓↓	↓↓↓	↓

↕ = $p < 0.05$ ↕↕ = $p < 0.01$ ↕↕↕ = $p < 0.001$ o = no significant change

– = not investigated

AT III = antithrombin III LDL = low-density lipoprotein HDL = high-density lipoprotein

By combining different forms of endocrine treatment the patient's tolerance of the therapy can be improved. CPA or small doses of OE alleviate the hot flushes after OR or during LHRH-A treatment, and blunt the initial rise in testosterone during treatment with LHRH-A [6, 13]. Furthermore, CPA induces certain metabolic changes opposite to those resulting from OE, and can thus be used to counteract side effects of OE [16–18, 22].

When selecting endocrine therapy for a particular patient it is essential to take into account the anticipated tolerance of the treatment with due respect to the patient's preference.

References

[1] Ahmed, S. R., J. B. F. Grant, S. M. Shalet et al.: A new hormonal therapy for prostatic cancer: Long-term clinical and hormonal response. Brit. J. Urol. **58** (1986) 534–538.

[2] Bergman, B., J.-E. Damber, B. Littbrand et al.: Sexual Function in Prostatic Cancer Patients Treated with Radiotherapy, Orchiectomy or Oestrogens. Brit. J. Urol. **56** (1984) 64–69.

[3] Blackard, C. E., R. P. Doe, G. T. Mellinger et al.: Incidence of cardiovascular disease and death in patients receiving diethylstilbestrol for carcinoma of the prostate. Cancer **26** (1970) 249–256.

[4] Blyth, B., C. U. McRae, E. A. Espiner et al.: Effect of stilboestrol on sodium balance, cardiac state, and renin-angiotensin-aldosterone activity in prostatic carcinoma. Brit. Med. J. **291** (1985) 1461–1464.

[5] de Voogt, H. J., P. H. Smith, M. Pavone-Macaluso et al.: Cardiovascular side effects of diethylstilbestrol, cyproterone acetate, medroxyprogesterone acetate and estramustin phosphate used for the treatment of advanced prostatic cancer: Results from European organization for research on treatment of cancer trials 30761 and 30762. J. Urol **135** (1986) 303–307.

[6] Eaton, A. C., N. McGuire: Cyproterone acetate in treatment of postorchidectomy hot flushes. Double-blind cross-over trial. Lancet **10** (1983) 1336–1337.

[7] Frödin, T., G. Ålund, E. Varenhorst: Measurement of skin bloodflow and water evaporation as a means of objectively assessing hot flushes after orchidectomy in patients with prostatic cancer. Prostate **7** (1985) 203–208.

[8] Glashan, R. W., M. R. G. Robinson: Cardiovascular Complications in the Treatment of Prostatic Carcinoma. Brit. J. Urol. **53** (1981) 624–627.

[9] Henriksson, P., O. Edhag: Orchidectomy versus oestrogen for prostatic cancer: cardiovascular effects. Brit. Med. J. **293** (1986) 413–415.

[10] Jacobi, G. H., J. E. Altwein, K. H. Kurth et al.: Treatment of Advanced Prostatic Cancer with Parenteral Cyproterone Acetate: A Phase III Randomised Trial. Brit. J. Urol. **52** (1980) 208–215.

[11] Paisey, R. B., C. Kadow, C. Bolton: Effects of cyproterone acetate and a long-acting LHRH analogue on serum lipoproteins in patients with carcinoma of the prostate. J. Roy. Soc. Med. **79** (1986) 210–211.

[12] Parmar, H., L. Edwards, R. H. Phillips et al.: Orchiectomy versus Long-acting D-Trp-6-LHRH in Advanced Prostatic Cancer. Brit. J. Urol. **59** (1987) 248–254.

[13] Svensson, M., E. Varenhorst, B. Kågedal: Initial administration of cyproterone acetate to prevent the rise of testosterone concentration during treatment with an LH-RH agonist in prostatic cancer. Anticancer Research **6** (1986) 379.

[14] Tveter, K. J., B. Otnes, R. Hannestad: Treatment of prostatic carcinoma with cyproterone acetate. Scand. J. Urol. Nephrol. **12** (1978) 115–118.

[15] Van Cangh, P. J., R. J. Opsomer. Treatment of advanced carcinoma of the prostate with a depot luteinizing hormone-releasing hormone analogue (ICI-118630). J. Urol. **137** (1987) 61–64.

[16] Varenhorst, E., B. E. Karlberg, L. Wallentin et al.: Effects of oestrogens, orchidectomy, and cyproterone acetate on salt and water metabolism in carcinoma of the prostate. Eur. Urol. 7 (1981) 231–236.

[17] Varenhorst, E., L. Wallentin, B. Risberg: The effects of orchidectomy, oestrogens, and cyproterone acetate on the antithrombin-III concentration in carcinoma of the prostate. Urol. Res. 9 (1981) 25–28.

[18] Varenhorst, E., B. Risberg: Effects of oestrogen, orchidectomy, and cyproterone acetate on tissue fibrinolysis in patients with carcinoma of the prostate. Invest. Urol. **18** (1981) 355–357.

[19] Varenhorst, E., G. Ålund, L. Wallentin et al.: Antithrombin III (AT III) und Plasmalipoproteine zur Beurteilung des kardiovaskulären Risikos während der Behandlung mit einem LH-RH-Agonisten bei Patienten mit Prostatakarzinom. Verhandlungsbericht der Deutschen Gesellschaft für Urologie **36** (1984) 581–582.

[20] Varenhorst, E., M. Svensson, H. Hjertberg et al.: Antithrombin III concentration, thrombosis, and treatment with luteinising hormone agonist in prostatic cancer. Brit. Med. J. **292** (1986) 935–936.

[21] Wallentin, L., E. Varenhorst: Plasma lipoproteins during treatment with cyproterone acetate in men with prostatic carcinoma. J. Clin. Endocrinol. Metab. **51** (1980) 1118–1122.

[22] Wallentin, L., E. Varenhorst: Plasma lipoproteins during antiandrogen treatment by oestrogens or orchidectomy in men with prostatic carcinoma. Horm. Metab. Res. **13** (1981) 293–297.

Result of long-term treatment with cyproterone acetate (CPA) in advanced prostatic cancer patients

F. Di Silverio, F. Sciarra

Introduction

Cyproterone acetate (CPA), a progestational compound displaying a potent antiandrogenic effect, has been used for many years for the treatment of advanced prostatic carcinoma (PC), with encouraging results. The drug possesses a dual action, not only inhibiting the gonadotropin secretion and testosterone production but also competing with androgens for receptor sites [9].

However CPA alone, at least in low dosage, is unable to induce the complete androgen neutralization in patients with PC: the remaining circulating androgens not only of testicular but also of adrenal origin, may therefore favour the evolution of the tumour, since it has been demonstrated that in milieu poor of androgens prostatic cancer cell may continue to grow, as a result of only 50% reduction of endogenous dihydrotestosterone (DHT) [4].

More favourable results can be obtained combining CPA treatment with bilateral orchiectomy, which completely inhibits the androgen action. Our experience on this combined treatment started in 1966 when orchiectomy was associated to CPA administered immediately after surgery or later in relation to the progression of the disease: from 1966 to 1975, 216 patients were treated by Bracci and Di Silverio following this protocol [1]. Successively CPA was administered by the group of Di Silverio [2, 3] only immediately after surgery and from 1976 to 1980 232 patients were followed. Finally from 1983 to 1986 53 patients were treated with CPA combined to a GnRH analogue (Zoladex) which induces a selective medical hypophysectomy and the block of the testicular secretion. In the present investigation, the results obtained in advanced PC treated with CPA immediately after surgical or medical castration are reported.

New Developments in Biosciences 4

Materials and methods

Two groups of patients affected by advanced PC, aged 54–86 years (mean 73 years), previously untreated were studied. The first group includes 232 patients treated with orchiectomy immediately combined to CPA (200 mg/die per os) with a follow-up of 60 months: 53 histologically graded G1, 94 G2 and 85 G3. 78 were in stage C and 154 in stage D, 127 of whom with bone metastases (D2). The second group includes 32 patients treated with Zoladex Depot (3.6 mg s. c. every 4 weeks) combined to CPA (200 mg/die): 2 histologically graded G1, 22 G2 and 8 G3. 22 were in stage C and 10 in stage D.

Hormonal investigations were determined in plasma samples taken at 8–9 a. m. before treatment and then 2 and 6 months after castration + CPA. In the cases treated with LH-RH-A + CPA hormonal assays were performed at the 3th–7th and 28th day after 9, 12 and 18 months. Gonadotropin LH-FSH, testosterone, androstenedione, dehydroepiandrosterone sulphate and prostatic acid phosphatase were determined by RIA [11].

The follow-up period ranged from 2 to 60 months. Criteria for determining the response to the endocrine therapy include the National Prostatic Cancer Project protocol; patients, showing remission or improvement of the subjective symptoms, regression of the tumour mass confirmed by ultrasonography and normalization of prostatic acid phosphatase were considered as having complete objective remission (COR) or partial objective regression (POR); patients showing clinical deterioration, increased size of tumour mass, pain, appearance of new metastases and increase in acid phosphatase were considered as having an objective progression (OP); finally patients presenting neither a clinical improvement nor a progression of the disease were considered objective stable (OS).

Results

Hormonal results

Treatment with orchiectomy + CPA: gonadotropins LH and FSH from pretreatment mean values of 14 $\pm$ 7.5 SD and 18 $\pm$ 5.5 mIU/ml rised after 1 months to 24.8 $\pm$ 14.8 and 27.5 $\pm$ 10.8 respectively ($p < 0.05$) showing a moderate increase to the end of the follow-up. On the contrary plasma T fall to castration values of 18.8 $\pm$ 8 ng/dl ($p < 0.001$) after 1 month, increased moderately to ng 30 $\pm$ 9.2 after 3 and 6 months and dropped again to the lowest values (18 ng/dl) thereafter. Plasma androstenedione decreased significantly from pre-treatment values of 133.5 $\pm$ 32 ng/dl to 45.6 $\pm$ 20 ng/dl ($p < 0.001$) and plasma DHEA.S from 1200 $\pm$ 240 ng/dl to 597 $\pm$ 156 ng/dl ($p < 0.001$).

Table 1 Zoladex + CPA treatment: clinical response

Months	3	(%)	6	(3)	9	(3)	12	(3)	18	(%)
COR	0/32	(0)	0/26	(0)	0/18	(0)	0/10	(0)	0/6	(0)
POR	24/32	(75)	22/26	(84.6)	16/18	(88.9)	10/10	(100)	6/6	(100)
OS	6/32	(18.8)	0/26	(0)	0/18	(0)	0/10	(0)	0/6	(0)
OP	2/32	(6.2)	4/26	(15.4)	2/18	(11.1)	0/10	(0)	0/6	(0)
number of patients	32		26		18		10		6	

Treatment with Zoladex + CPA: during the first week of therapy LH and FSH did not change significantly with respect to pre-treatment values, but after 1 month LH decreased to 7.5 ± 3.1 mIU/ml, remaining at about 4.5 ± 2.3 ($p < 0.01$) up to end of the follow-up which was 18 months; FSH remained around 6.1 ± 2.6 mIU/ml. Plasma T showed no significant changes during the first week of therapy but dropped after the first month to 25 ± 6 ng/dl ($p < 0.01$), whilst DHEA.S decreased from 1180 ± 490 ng/ml to 711 ± 200 ng/ml ($p < 0.01$).

Clinical results

In stage C – D PC, the survival rate following orchiectomy + CPA administration decreases progressively from 83% after 1 year to 66% after 3 years, but after 72 months 58% of the patients are still alive (fig. 1). Comparing the results obtained in 27 patients in stage D2 immediately treated with CPA after castration with those of 26 patients in stage D2 in whom CPA was given later, in progression of the disease, it can be seen that the survival rate is improved significantly ($p < 0.05$) in the first group: 62% being still alive after 36 months (fig. 2). 3 out of 4 G1 were in progression 8, 13 and 18 months respectively after castration, 8 out of 13 G2 were in progression between 2 and 12 months and 9 out of 9 G3 were in progression between 1 and 12 months.

The survival rate is higher in stage C PC, being 66% of the patients still alive after 72 months treatment. 78% of the patients showed a marked reduction of the primary tumour after 3 months of combined therapy, confirmed by T. R. sonography. In 72% of 127 patients in stage D2 complete or partial relief of pain was observed. PAP levels decreased from mean values of 10 ng/ml to 2 – 3 ng/ml, remaining around these values up to 60 months of treatment.

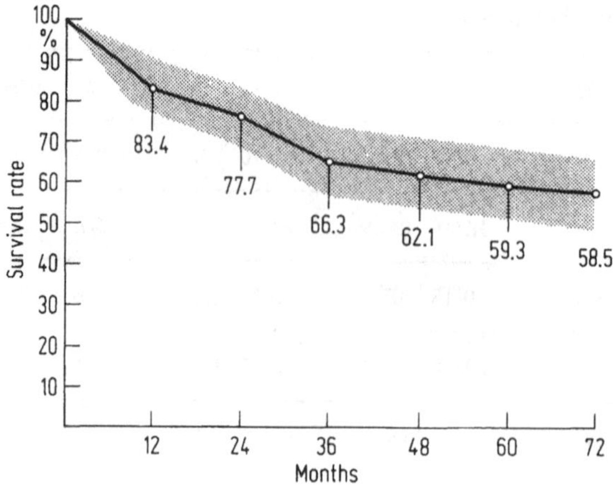

Fig. 1 Stage C + D: Survival rate following orchiectomy + CPA (200 mg/day). (Number of patients = 232)

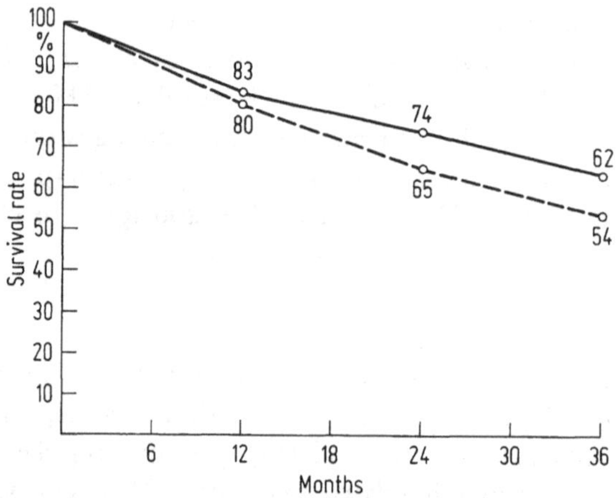

Fig. 2 Stage D2: Survival rate following
orchiectomy + CPA (immediatly) ——— (n = 27)
orchiectomy + CPA (given later) - - - - (n = 26).
($p < 0.05$)

As far as the medical castration with Zoladex Depot combined to CPA, after 3 months 24 out of 32 patients were in POR, 2 in OP (both G2 stage D) and the remaining cases in OS. After 6 months 22 out of 26 patients were in POR and 4 in OP (2 G2 and 2 G3, 2 stage C and 2 stage D) whilst after 9 months 16 out of 18 were in POR and 2 in OP (both G3, stage C). At the 12th and 18th month all patients, 10 and 6 respectively, were in POR (tab. 1). 38.4% of the patients in stage D showed a marked reduction of the primary tumour, but 46% showed no modification and 15.5% presented an increase in tumour size. A marked reduction of the metastases was observed only in 7.7% of the cases, whereas in 61.5% no modification and in 30.8% progressive deterioration was seen. Bone pain disappeared in 27.3% of the cases, remained unchanged in 54.5% and increased in 18.2%. PAP levels decreased form mean values of 17 ng/ml to 3 ng/ml, remaining around 1 – 5 ng/ml up to the 18th month of follow-up.

Discussion

In advanced PC, treatment with CPA combined to medical or surgical castration, induces significant hormonal changes, with a complete neutralization of the androgen action: plasma testosterone drops to very low levels comparable to those of the normal women, as a result of the peripheral conversion from adrenal precursors. But also the adrenal androgens undergo a significant decrease since CPA possesses also a suppressive effect on the adrenocorticotropic hormones [5]. This effect is very important since adrenal androgens may be peripherally transformed into strong androgens, which may be utilized by the PC tissue. In fact measurement of prostatic concentrations of DHT following castration shows that the adrenal contribution to DHT formation may be evaluated around 40% [4]. Furthermore it has been demonstrated that low serum androgen levels, still present in castrated patients, are sufficient to stimulate PC growth [10].

From a clinical point of view, it has been demonstrated that the combined treatment orchiectomy + CPA, started immediately after diagnosis, gives remission in almost 80% of the cases increasing the survival up to 72 months in 58% of the patients. Therefore, orchiectomy alone should not be performed any more on account the higher incidence of mortality during the first 1 – 2 years.

The clinical improvement is rapid: pain disappeares within few days and the urinary symptoms decrease in 3 months. Appetite and body weight increase progressively so that most of the patients return to normal life activities.

A true alternative to surgical castration is represented by the treatment with LH-RH analogues, that avoid the psycological implication of orchiectomy. Androgen activity is constantly suppressed and the combination therapy with CPA prevents the T rise during the first days of treatment which could result in a flare-up of the clinical situation. Moreover adrenal androgens are neutralized. A combined treatment with LHRH analogues and antiandrogens as flutamide or anandron has been performed also by Labrie et al., who observed a positive response in 100% of the cases [7, 8]. Other investigators, however, did not obtain convincing results [6]. These discrepancies in our opinion, can be clarified increasing the follow-up period on a larger group of patients, possibly in multicenter randomized studies.

Conclusion

CPA has be employed in association with surgical or medical castration, for the complete neutralization of the androgen action.

- CPA has to be used immediately after orchiectomy or combined to LHRH analogues and not later during the progression of the disease or discontinuously.
- The oral dosage is 200 mg/day.
- Side effects are lower than those observed with other antiandrogens or estrogens.
- CPA is the antiandrogen of first choice.

References

[1] Bracci, U.: Our present procedure in the treatment of prostatic cancer. In: U. Bracci, F. Di Silverio (eds.): Hormonal therapy of prostatic cancer, pp. 177 – 192. Cofese Palermo 1, 1975.

[2] Di Silverio, F., F. Sciarra, F. Piro et al.: Testosterone totale, testosterone liberio, diidrotestosterone e SHBH nel carcinoma della prostata: modificazioni indotte dalla orchiectomia e dal ciproterone acetato. LI Cong. Soc. It. Urol., Trieste sept. 1978. C. Corbi (ed.), pp. 1 – 10. Cofese Palermo, 1978.

[3] Di Silverio, F., F. Sciarra, C. Piro: Effetto della orchiectomia, del ciproterone acetato e dell'orchiectomia più ciproterone acetato sui valori plasmatici del testosterone totale, testosterone libero, diidrotestosterone e sex hormone binding globulin in pazienti con carcinoma prostatico. Rivista Oncologia, 3 (1980) 165 – 174.

[4] Geller, J., J. Albert, S. S. C. Yen: Treatment of advanced cancer of the prostate with megestrol acetate. Urol. 12 (1978) 537 – 541.

[5] Girard, J., J. B. Baumann, U. Buhler et al.: Cyproterone acetate and ACTH adrenal function. J. Clin. Endocr. Metab. 47 (1978) 581.

[6] Giuliani, L., T. Barreca, C. Giberti et al.: Treatment of prostatic cancer with a depot form of a luteinizing hormone-releasing hormone. Europ. Journ. 12 (6) (1986) 390 – 394.

[7] Labrie, F., A. Dupont, A. Belanger et al.: New approach in the treatment of prostate cancer: complete instead of only partial withdrawal of androgens. Prostate 4 (1983) 579 – 594.

[8] Labrie, F., A. Dupont, A. Belanger: New hormonal therapy in prostatic carcinoma: combined treatment with LHRH agonist and an antiandrogen. J. Clin. Invest. Med. 5 (1982) 267 – 275.

[9] Neumann, F., K. J. Graf, S. H. Hason et al.: Central actions of antiandrogens. In: L. Martini, M. Motta (eds.): Androgens and antiandrogens, pp. 163 – 171. Raven Press, New York 1977.

[10] Stoliar, B., D. J. Albert: SCH 13521 in the treatment of advanced carcinoma of the prostate. J. Urol. 111 (1974) 803 – 807.

[11] Toscano, V., E. Petrangeli, M. V. Adamo et al.: Simultaneous determination of 5 alfa-reduced metabolites of testosterone in human plasma. J. Steroid Biochem. 6 (1981) 574 – 578.

Results and experience with the androgen ablation therapy: current trends in the USA

D. Kirchheim

Introduction

Hormonal therapy of prostatic cancer was recognized and initiated by Huggins and Hodges in 1941 [8]. Prior to the "hormonal area", only complications of prostatic cancer were treated by medications or surgical relief of urinary obstruction. Bumpus from the Mayo Clinic increased the five-year survival rate by suprapubic cystostomy in 1926 from 10 percent to 36 percent [4]. In the mid-thirties the introduction of sulfonamides by Domagk further improved the quality of life of prostatic cancer patients. Nesbit and Baum [13] published their larger series of hormonally treated prostatic cancer patients. The best results of 44 percent five-year survival rates were achieved with initial bilateral orchiectomy followed by a daily dosage of 5 mg of Stilbestrol. Since Young's first publication on total (radical) prostatectomy in 1905, an increasing number of American urologists advised early diagnosis of prostatic cancer by annual rectal examinations in men over fifty years to try to cure the cancer by complete surgical excision. In the sixties, Bagshaw and other radiotherapists [1, 5] devised high dosage radiation techniques to destroy or arrest prostatic cancer cells. Hormonal therapy became the domain of patients with advanced prostatic cancer or older patients with a less than ten year expected survival prognosis.

Many different estrogenic substances in variables dosages have been tried out. Twelve medical institutions in the United States undertook a cooperative study of various hormonal treatments and dosages *after* relapse of prostatic cancer patients who had initially been treated with orchiectomy. Neither 5 mg nor 500 mg of Stilbestrol daily showed no response and no statistically different results. Testosterone showed in some instances exacerbation ("flare") of the cancer or no effect. Prednisone and medroxyprogesterone showed no significant benefits [6].

Andrenalectomy [3, 7] or medical adrenalectomy with cortisone or other adrenal inhibiting drugs were tried around the fifties and later, to eliminate also the androgens from the adrenal glands after orchiectomy had failed ("total androgen blockage"). Because of no significant improvement, these procedures were even-

New Developments in Biosciences 4

tually abandoned. For similar reasons, hypophysectomy was carried out [3, 16]. Chiefly for relief of intolerable pain, not relieved by other means, it is now done by transphenoidal approach with low morbidity.

Hodges and Kirchheim [6] reviewed the state of hormonal management in 1967: Orchiectomy was a standard therapy. Stilbestrol (or other estrogens) only acted by inhibition of pituitary gonadotrophins ("medical orchiectomy") and had no proven direct effect on the prostatic cancer cells [10, 15].

Between 1961 and 1967, sixteen Veterans Hospitals, including the urological teaching service of the V. A. Hospital in Portland, Oregon, undertook the well-known VACURG prostatic cancer studies comprising over 2000 patients. Most of their results were published between 1967 and 1973 [2, 18].

Initially the results published in 1967 showed similar survival rates for placebo and orchiectomy and estrogens, which was difficult to conceive. Actually, we physician investigators treated patients randomized into the placebo group eventually with Stilbestrol or orchiectomy for medical ethical reasons when they began to become symptomatic or their clinical condition deteriorated. However, our statisticians still carried these patients in the placebo group. Eventually these misunderstandings were corrected and in spite of it, significant conclusions were arrived at:

1. Bilateral orchiectomy or Stilbestrol were more effective than placebo in delaying the progression of prostatic carcinoma from Stage C (regional) to Stage D (metastatic).
2. Early hormonal treatment of prostatic cancer did not increase the survival time versus therapy in later stages of prostatic cancer (symptomatic or metastatic).
3. Patients treated with 5 mg Stilbestrol had a higher mortality and morbidity from cardiovascular diseases than patients treated by bilateral orchiectomy.

Since then we have tried to limit the side-effects of estrogens by giving the lowest dosage which achieves anorchid levels. Most of our patients have been treated with 1 mg Stilbestrol daily. We advise pre-treatment radiation to the male breast tissue to avoid gynecomastia and nipple soreness. We recommend to patients with cardiovascular disease bilateral orchiectomy or Luteinizing hormone releasing hormone agonists (LHRH). Antiandrogens are presently not available in the United States, except in clinical trials.

If patients show relapse (clinical deterioration or other evidence of disease progression) we check serum testosterone levels. If they are not at anorchid levels, orchiectomy is recommended. We have had a few of our patients on intermittent 1 mg daily Stilbestrol therapy with resumption of potency and no change in the course of their illness for longer intervals. Klotz et al. [11] reported a series of patients on intermittent endocrine therapy for advanced prostatic cancer.

Patients and type of study

1012 patients with a diagnosis of prostatic cancer have been treated at St. Peter Hospital in Olympia, Washington or in our outpatient clinic between 1973 and 1984. 225 patients were treated initially by hormonal manipulations (estrogens or bilateral orchiectomy). 48 patients were excluded from the study: 28 because of inadequate follow-up or noncompliance with treatment, 13 because of other cancers – chiefly colon, lung, and brain, and seven because of phlebitis or pulmonary emboli following Stilbestrol therapy. 177 patients had satisfactory follow-up and comprise this study.

Results

Our clinical results are shown in figures 1 and 2. Seventy-six of the 177 hormonally treated patients were clinically diagnosed as Stage C (regional). Many of these tumors consisted of larger volumes (over 25 to 80 grams) and had proportionately a higher likelihood of showing at least microscopic lymphnode metastases if retropubic lymphnode resections would have been done.

The 10 year survival rate of the Stilbestrol (D. E. S.) treated and orchiectomized Stage C patients was over 10 percent (fig. 1). The five year survival of the Stilbestrol treated patients was 56 percent. However, the five year survival of the orchiectomized Stage C patients was only 27 percent. Further analysis of our records suggested that this was due to the fact that the number in this group was small (n = 20) and six patients died within the first four years from other causes.

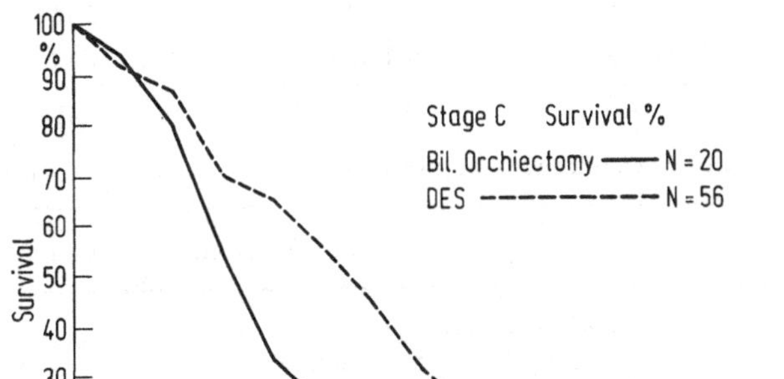

Fig. 1 Survival rates of patients with stage C (T 3 or T 4, MO) Prostatic Cancer.

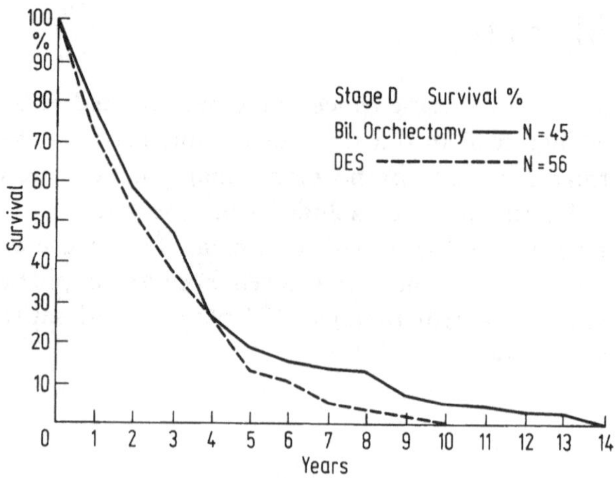

Fig. 2 Survival rates of patients with stage D (T 2–4, N+ M+) Prostatic Cancer.

Figure 2 shows the survival rate of 101 patients with *metastatic* prostatic cancer disease. The 45 orchiectomized patients had a slightly better and longer survival than the Stilbestrol treated patients. Considering other factors such as tumor volume, grade of differentiation and age of patient at the beginning of treatment, there was no statistically significant difference.

Fifty percent of the orchiectomized patients were still alive at two years and 10 months and eight percent at 10 years. The most dramatic and important effects were improvement in the quality of life, relief of pain and general and functional recovery in over 80 percent of the patients.

We recommend bilateral orchiectomy especially in patients with bone metastases and symptoms as first choice. It is a short minor surgical procedure usually performed as an outpatient. Loss of potency and hot flashes are the main side

Table 1 Side effects and complications of androgen ablations therapy

	Orchiectomy	Estrogens*	LHRH agon.	Antiandrogens
Cardiovascular	–	+ +	–	–
Impotence	+ +	+ +	+ +	–
Gynecomastia	–	+ +	–	+
Hot flashes	+ +	–	+	–
Tumor flare	–	–	+	–
Gastrointestinal	–	–/+	–	–/+
Minor Surgery	+	–	–	–

* dose dependent

effects (tab. 1). If the patient does not accept orchiectomy, mostly for psychological reasons or rarely has medical contraindications, Stilbestrol is recommended. Most patients were started on 1 mg Stilbestrol twice daily for a month and then maintained on 1 mg D. E. S. daily. If nipple soreness or gynecomastia occurs or the patient does not respond to therapy, serum testosterone levels are determined. Our goal is to decrease serum testosterone levels close to anorchid values. Using the lowest effective dosage.

Discussion

Table 1 shows the side effects of various types of hormonal therapies. Luteinizing hormone releasing hormone (LHRH) agonists may become more readily accepted when it can be given by longer acting drugs intramuscularly at monthly or longer intervals. As for antiandrogens (cyproterone acetate, flutamide) these are presently not yet available for clinical use in the United States. If these drugs have lesser side effects than Stilbestrol and other estrogens, they would become another alternative.

Clinical and research investigations [12, 14] show that the human prostate is not responsive to *adrenal* androgens. Eventually prostatic cancer cell populations become refractory to androgen ablation therapy and further hormonal therapies show no significant statistical results after primary proper hormonal therapy fails [9]. Research priorities may be better directed towards diagnostic methods to recognize hormonally non-responsive prostatic cancers [17] and initiate earlier and more effective chemotherapies.

Summary

The evolution of hormonal treatment since its introduction by Huggins and Hodges in 1941 is critically reviewed. In a 12-year period (1973 to 1984) 1012 patients with prostatic cancer were seen. Of 225 patients initially treated with hormonal therapy, 177 fulfilled the criteria for this clinical study. Of the 76 patients diagnosed clinically as Stage C, 56 percent Stilbestrol treated patients survived five years and more than 10 percent ten years. Of the 101 patients diagnosed with metastases (Stage D) 50 percent of the orchiectomized patients were alive at two years and eight months and eight percent at 10 years. Based on our present knowledge we start hormonal therapy when the patient shows evidence of metastases or becomes significantly symptomatic. Bilateral orchiectomy was the most reliable therapy with the least side effects. Patients who declined orchiectomy mostly for psychological reasons or had medical contra indications were treated with Stilbestrol (D. E. S.). In order to minimize estrogenic side effects, our goal was to use the lowest possible dosage of Stilbestrol to decrease serum testosterone levels close to anorchid values. In the majority of patients, 1 mg Stilbestrol as a daily dosage was sufficient.

References

[1] Bagshaw, M. A.: Radiation therapy of prostatic carcinoma. In: E. D. Crawford, T. A. Borden (eds.): Genitourinary Cancer Surgery, pp. 405–411. Lea & Febiger, Philadelphia 1986.
[2] Blackard, C. I., D. P. Byar, W. P. Jordan et al.: Orchiectomy for advanced prostatic cancer, a reevaluation. Urology **1** (1973) 553–559.
[3] Brendler, H.: Adrenalectomy and hypophysectomy for prostatic cancer. Urology **2** (1973) 99–105.
[4] Bumpus, H. C.: Surg. Gynec. & Obst. **43** (1926) 154–160.
[5] Del Regato, J. A.: Radiotherapy in the conservative treatment of operable and locally inoperable carcinoma of the prostate. Radiology **88** (1967) 761–766.
[6] Hodges, C. V., D. Kirchheim: Hormone treatment of cancer of the prostate. In: G. Rentchnik (ed.): Cancer results in cancer research, pp. 133–142, 1967.
[7] Huggins, C., D. M. Bergenstal: Surgery of the adrenals. J. A. M. A. **147** (1951) 101–106.
[8] Huggins, C., C. V. Hodges: Studies on prostatic cancer: effect of castration, of estrogen and of androgen injection on serum phosphatases in metastatic carcinoma of the prostate. Cancer Res. **1** (1941) 293–297.
[9] Isaacs, J. T., D. S. Coffey: Adaptation versus selection as the mechanism responsible for the relapse of prostatic cancer to androgen ablation therapy as studied in the Dunning R-3327-H adenocarcinoma. Cancer Res. **41** (1981) 5070–5075.
[10] Kirchheim, D., W. W. Scott: The effects of castration and sex hormones upon aminopeptidases and phosphatases of the rat prostate. Invest. Urol. **2** (1965) 393–404.
[11] Klotz, L. H., M. W. Herr, M. J. Morse et al.: Intermittent endocrine therapy of advanced prostate cancer. Cancer **58** (1966) 2546–2550.
[12] Lepor, H., A. Ross, P. C. Walsh: The influence of hormonal therapy on survival of men with advanced prostatic cancer. J. Urol. **128** (1922) 335–340.
[13] Nesbit, R. M., W. C. Baum: Endocrine control of prostatic carcinoma. J. A. M. A. **113** (1950) 1317–1320.
[14] Oesterling, J. E., J. I. Epstein, P. C. Walsh: The inability of adrenal androgens to stimulate the adult human prostate: an autopsy evaluation of men with hypogonadotrophic hypogonadism and panhypopituitarism. J. Urol. **126** (1986).
[15] Rothauge, C. F., O. Weller, E. Schuchardt: Die Wirkung von Diathyldioxystilben-diphosphat (Honvan®) auf die Keimdrüse und die Gonadotropinausscheidung beim Manne. Klin. Wschr. **41** (1963) 90–95.
[16] Scott, W. W., H. K. A. Schirmer: Hypophysectomy for disseminated prostate cancer. In: Essays in experimenta biology, pp. 175–182, Univ. of Chicago Press, Chicago 1962.
[17] Trachtenberg, J., P. C. Walsh: Correlation of prostatic nuclear androgen receptor content with duration of response and survival following hormonal therapy in advanced prostatic cancer. J. Urol. **127** (1982) 466–473.
[18] Veterans Administration Cooperative Urological Research Group: Treatment and survival of patients with cancer of the prostate. Surg. Gynec. & Obst. **124** (1967) 1011–1017.

Long-term results of an LH-RH agonist monotherapy in patients with carcinoma of the prostate and reflections on the so-called total androgen blockade with pre-medicated cyproterone acetate

G. H. Jacobi

Introduction

Shortly after it had been found out that synthetic analogues of the genuine LH-releasing hormone (LH-RH analogues or LH-RH agonists), if applied in "supra-physiological" doses and in continuous succession, act to suppress testosterone down to the castrate level, this principle of action was introducted into the so-called contrasexual therapy of the metastasizing carcinoma of the prostate [7, 15]. Meanwhile, several LH-RH agonists have been commercialized, either for pernasal (buserelin), subcutaneous (buserelin, Leuprolide, Decapeptyl®) or for intramusucular (Decapeptyl® Depot) application. Other depot forms of these analogue hormones (buserelin, Zoladex) are at the present time the object of world-wide experimental and clinical studies.

Our present knowledge – based on six years of clinical research on patients with an advanced carcinoma of the prostate – permits the conclusion that all above mentioned LH-RH agonists are equally effective in their castrative effect, clinical potency and their low incidence of tolerable side effects. Advantages or disadvantages, if there are any, only concern the costs of treatment, the various forms of application and the resulting different degrees of compliance.

This clinic has been engaged in intensive animal experiments and clinical trials with the LH-RH analogues buserelin (Suprefact®) and Decapeptyl® (Decapeptyl® Depot) since October, 1981. A randomized therapy study has been under way for three years now in cooperation with the European Organisation for Research on Treatment of Cancer (E. O. R. T. C.: de Voogt, Amsterdam; Klijn, Rotterdam).

New Developments in Biosciences 4

Buserelin or Decapeptyl® Depot as a monotherapy

Between October, 1981, and September, 1987, more than 200 patients with an advanced carcinoma of the prostate have been treated in this clinic. The present long-term analysis of the results comprises 151 patients (122 treated with buserelin and 29 with Decapeptyl® Depot).

85 patients from the buserelin-treated group and 22 patients from the Decapeptyl®-Depot-treated group are at our disposal with a follow-up period of at least 18 months duration.

Table 1 shows the different dosage schemes for both LH-RH analogues. Over the last two years buserelin was applied only pernasally at a continuous dose of 3 × 300 μg/day.

Table 1 Dosage schemes for pernasal and subcutaneous buserelin and intramuscular Decapeptyl®-Depot

Dose Regimen

Buserelin	– 2 × 200 μg/d s.c. 14 days	and 3 × 400 μg/d p.n. thereafter
	– 3 × 1000 μg/d s.c. 6 days	
	– 3 × 500 μg/d s.c. 6 days	
	– 3 × 300 μg/d p.n. contineously	
Decapeptyl®	– D-Trp 6-LHRH 3.2 mg microencapsulated in 119 mg Lyophilisate injected i.m. every 5 weeks	

All patients had an advanced cancer of the prostate with no preceding therapy. The age of the patients varied between 49 and 86 years (average: 70 years). 76 patients had a carcinoma category M_1 with distant metastases (71 p.c.), whereas 31 patients (29 p.c.) suffered from an advanced locoregional carcinoma of the tumour category T_3 N_X M_O. All patients showed measurable tumour lesions to evaluate an objective tumour regression by means of computerized tomography, sonography and X-ray diagnosis. All patients were checked through repeated skeleton scans. Further controls in all patients covered such laboratory parameters as the prostate-specific phosphatase and the prostate-specific antigen (since 1984).

Results

Figure 1 shows the long-term testosterone curve and the behaviour of LH basal and after stimulation for the buserelin group. A short stimulation phase between days 3 and 7 of treatment – with the testosterone values rising from 4.8 ± 2.2 ng/ml to 6.5 ± 2.4 ng/ml – is followed by a down regulation, which after four

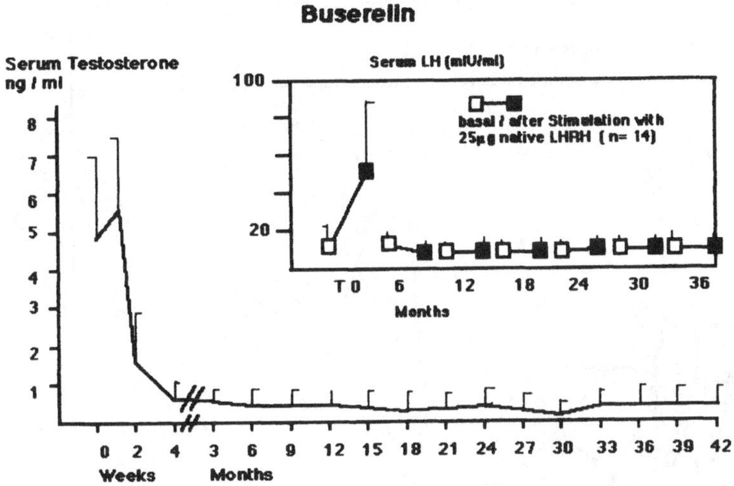

Fig. 1 Serum testosterone curve (mean values ± standard deviation) in 85 patients on a buserelin monotherapy; the inset shows the results of the LH-RH stimulation test for 14 patients.

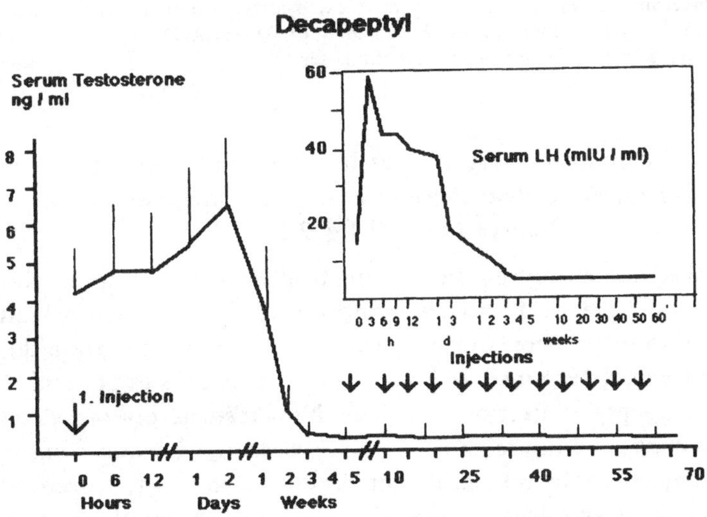

Fig. 2 Serum testosterone curve (mean values ± standard deviation) in 22 patients on a Decapeptyl® Depot monotherapy; the inset shows the serum LH curve for the same group of patients.

weeks leads to castrate values for serum testosterone (0.5 ng/ml). As long as treatment continues, the serum testosterone remains at the castrate level. At the same time the stimulability of LH ceases in spite of the administration of 25 µg of native LH-RH (inset of fig. 1).

The injection of Decapeptyl® Depot at intervals of 5 weeks gives a comparable testosterone curve (fig. 2) with stimulation-induced values from 4.5 ±1.2 ng/ml

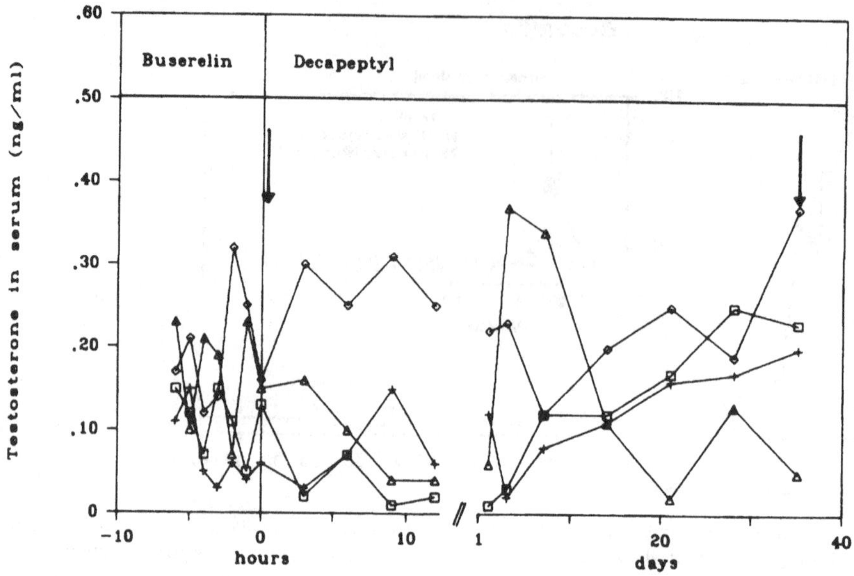

Fig. 3 Serum testosterone curves of 4 patients prior to, and after, switching over from 3 × 300 μg of buserelin a day pernasally to injections of 3.2 mg of Devapeptyl® Depot (DTrp-6-LH-RH) i.m. once every 5 weeks; for further explanations see text.

initially to 6.3 ± 1.8 ng/ml on day 2 after injection and a down regulation to castrate levels after no more than three weeks. The testosterone curve is amply parallelled by the serum LH curve (inset of fig. 2).

Four patients asked for a continuation of medication with intramuscular injections of Decapeptyl® Depot 11 to 26 months (average: 18 months) after the pernasal buserelin therapy. After the last pernasal buserelin application the serum testosterone level was determined at hourly intervals over 6 hours and the first intramuscular Decapeptyl® injection was given. Now testosterone was determined at 3-hour intervals over 12 hours and then weekly. As can be seen from figure 3, this therapy change brought no significant difference in the testosterone down regulation: the testosterone levels remained in all patients at the castrate level (under 0.5 ng/ml). All patients retained the condition of an objective remission.

To evaluate the clinical response to the buserelin or Decapeptyl® Depot therapy, we first applied the response criteria of the E. O. R. T. C. and compared the data obtained with the criteria of the National Prostatic Cancer Treatment Group (NPCTG). The clinical response was evaluated six months after commencement of treatment. The patients treated with buserelin, had a follow-up period of 2 to 4.5 years, those treated with Decapeptyl® one of 15 to 24 months. Table 2 shows the response data under the E. O. R. T. C. criteria, whereas table 3 gives a comparison of the clinical response rates. The average response time (partial or

Table 2 Clinical response rates (evaluation after 6 months) in 107 patients on a monotherapy with LH-RH agonists

Clinical Response (E. O. R. T. C. Criteria)		
Objective	Buserelin (n = 85)	Decapeptyl® (n = 22)
Partial and complete response	54%	51%
No change	25%	33%
Progression	21%	16%
Subjective	25/31 (81%)	7/9 (78%)

Table 3 Comparison between the clinical response rates (107 patients from table 2) under the criteria of the E. O. R. T. C. and the National Prostatic Cancer Treatment Group (N. P. C. T. G.); it should be recalled that the category "stable disease" of the N. P. C. T. G. is rated as a therapy success, whereas the category "no change" of the E. O. R. T. C. is rated as a therapy failure.

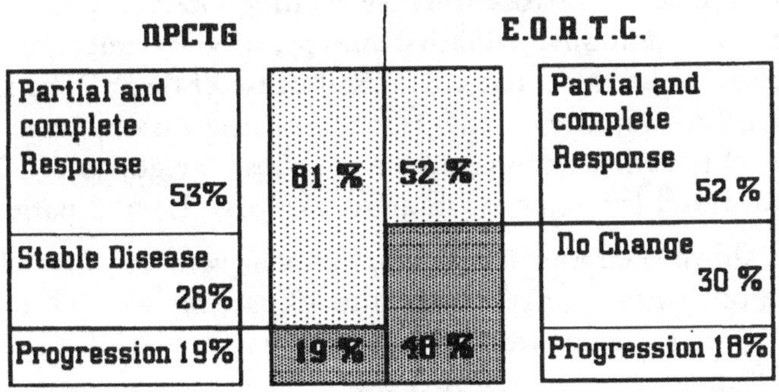

complete remission) is 23 months for the buserelin-treated patients, and 14 months for the Decapeptyl® Depot group. The subjective response to the therapy was determined two months after commencement of treatment; 32 out of 40 patients with osseous metastases reported a significant reduction of pain.

Relapses after buserelin

The remission rate of 54 p.c. after buserelin (table 2) is based on a six-month follow-up regime. However out of the entire group of the patients treated since 1981 46 showed a relapse after a primary partial or complete remission. These patients have meanwhile been in the follow-up regime for 30 to 58 months, which

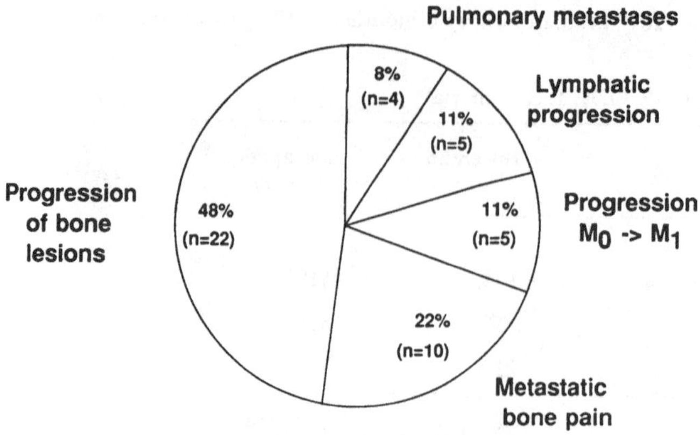

Fig. 4 First sign of the relapse in 46 patients on a buserelin monotherapy after a primary partial or complete remission; the 10 patients with pain from osseous metastases had skeletal metastases already initially and were free from pain during the objective remission phase.

covers the following parameters: first objective sign of the secondary progression, correlation of the initial serum testosterone levels, time interval until the occurrence of the progression, additional palliative therapy, survival time, time interval between occurrence of progression and death, and cause of death. The indicator lesions, which helped to objectivate the secondary progression, were osseous metastases (M_1) in 39 patients, lymph node metastases (categories N_2, N_4) in 4 patients, and the advanced locoregional tumour (category T_4) in 3 patients.

In 36 patients the above mentioned indicator lesions were the first clue of a progression in need of treatment, as compared to 10 patients where the progression was signalled by major pains from osseous metastases (fig. 4).

The time interval until the occurrence of the progression reaches from 3 to 45 months (average: 13.6 months). 32 patients (70 p.c.) died: 31 from cancer of the prostate, one from a myocardial infarction [8].

The time interval from the objectivated secondary progression to death was between 0 and 30 months (average: 10.5 months), the survival time reached from 3 to 58 months (average: 27 months). At the time of the progression 36 patients, while continuing the buserelin therapy, were treated with additional palliative measures: high-dosed i.v. fosfestrol therapy (Honvan®, 12 g/10 days) and/or estramustine phosphate (31 patients); local radiotherapy of painful skeleton regions (5 patients); systemic therapy with the radioisotope yttrium (9 patients).

To find out up to which degree the initial androgen balance of the patients may have an impact on the long-term results of the medicamentous castration by means of LH-RH agonists, we correlated the response rates to the initial (pretherapy) serum testosterone differentiating between patients with normal serum testosterone levels (avove 2.5 ng/ml) and patients with an initial serum testosterone below this lower limit. 14 of the 46 patients with a secondary relapse (30.4 p.c.) had subnormal pre-therapy testosterone levels, which had, however, no influence on the time interval of the clinical response (time until progression): this was 13.6 months for all 46 patients, 14.2 months for patients with an initially normal testosterone level, and 12.5 months for those with an initially subnormal testosterone level. This result is in contradiction with a study by Hickey et al. [6] based on a heterogenous material as far as the contrasexual therapy forms are concerned. These authors observed no objective tumour regression in any of the patients with an initial serum testosterone under 2.0 ng/ml, although the pre-therapy testosterone levels were not significantly different in the groups with a clinical response or a therapy failure.

Total androgen blockade

The rational basis for the additional suppression of the residual androgens after orchiectomy or a contrasexual therapy with LH-RH agonists (testosterone lower than 0.5 ng/ml) at the target organ by antiandrogens is seen in the hypothesis by Labrie et al. [10], according to which adrenal androgens cumulate in the carcinoma of the prostate as dihydrotestosterone thus stimulating the further growth of the carcinoma. Furthermore, an additional testosterone-dependent proliferation of the carcinoma of the prostate is supposed to set in the initial stimulation phase of the LH-RH agonist therapy (figs. 1 and 2).

This problem lies in the centre of an E. O. R. T. C. protocol (30843), which was initiated in 1984 (fig. 5). Patients with an untreated carcinoma of the prostate with distant metastases were randomly distributed over three therapy groups:

1. bilateral orchiectomy as a so-called reference therapy;

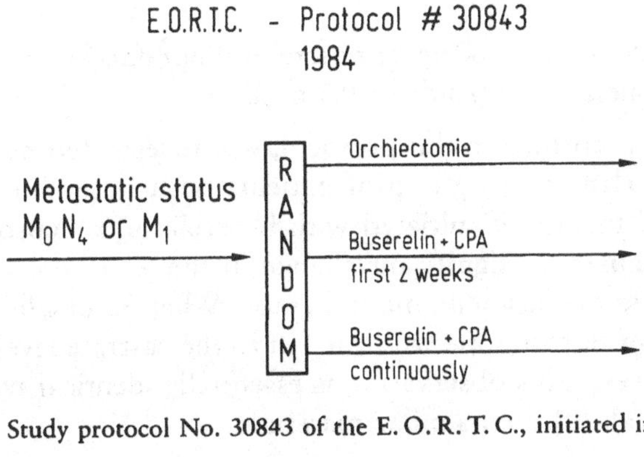

Fig. 5 Study protocol No. 30843 of the E. O. R. T. C., initiated in 1984.

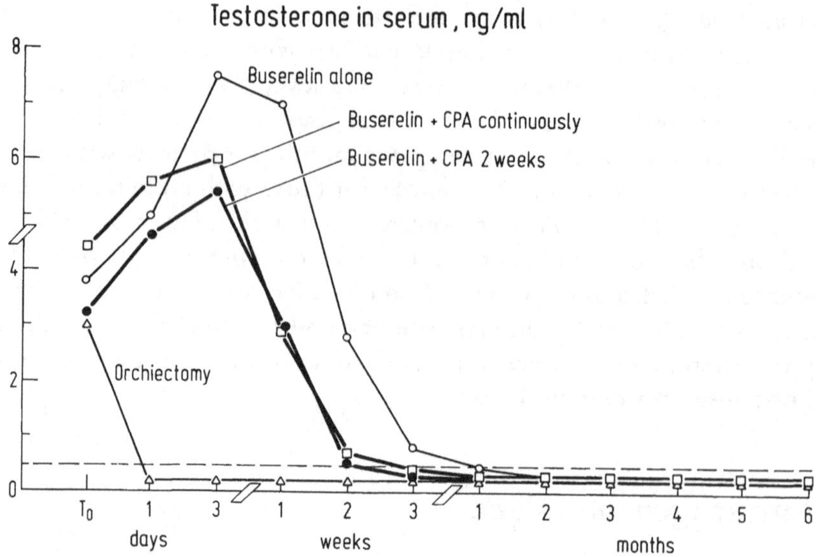

Fig. 6 Serum testosterone curves of the following groups of patients:
64 patients with a buserelin monotherapy (historic control group),
8 patients with buserelin plus cyproterone acetate (CPA) continuously,
8 patients with buserelin plus CPA over two weeks,
7 patients with a bilateral orchiectomy.

2. buserelin for "medicamentous castration", combined with the antiandrogen cyproterone acetate over the first two weeks of therapy, followed by a buserelin monotherapy. This branch of therapy has the purpose of suppressing the testosterone stimulation phase of the first two weeks by the action of the antiandrogen;
3. buserelin plus cyproterone acetate as a continuous combined therapy (so-called total androgen blockade). This branch of therapy has the purpose of measuring the impact of the residual adrenal androgens (after castration) on the clinical response.

The daily doses in this study are 3 × 400 µg of buserelin (Suprefact®) pernasally, and 3 × 50 mg of cyproterone acetate (Androcur®) orally.

We have treated 23 patients according to this protocol, whose testosterone curves are compared in figure 6 to an earlier group of patients on a buserelin monotherapy. If the contrasexual therapy is initiated with buserelin plus cyproterone acetate, the antiandrogen causes no significant change in the testosterone stimulation phase, as compared to the buserelin monotherapy. What occurs, however, is a faster down regulation of testosterone with the fall to the castrate level being anticipated by about one week. This observation is essentially identical with the results obtained by Klijn et al. [9] on a similar material.

But if the two therapy components of the total androgen blockade (LH-RH agonist plus antiandrogens) set in with a time lag between them, the testosterone stimulation phase of the LH-RH agonists can be modulated. Svensson et al. [13] gave their prostate cancer patients a 15-day pre-treatment with cyproterone acetate thus achieving as significant diminution of serum testosterone and an intracellular blockade of the action of androgens. The following additional therapy with the LH-RH agonist Zoladex did produce a transitory testosterone stimulation with a peak on day 4, but the testosterone levels failed to reach the pre-therapy range. The castrate level for testosterone was reached a fortnight after the first Zoladex Depot implanation and was maintained after the second implanation four weeks later – in spite of the discontinuation of cyproterone acetate. Boccon-Gibod et al. [1] attained almost identical results in a 7-day therapeutic pre-medication phase with cyproterone acetate and a subsequent additonal therapy with the LH-RH agonist buserelin, as did Urwin et al. [14] with cyproterone acetate plus Zoladex.

Habenicht et al. [5] investigated this phenomenon in more detail on young healthy volunteers. Those authors demonstrated the LH-RH agonist-induced testosterone suppression of stimulation with a pre-medicated antiandrogen in the same group of volunteers. These were treated at first with buserelin (3 × 500 µg s.c./day) over 7 days, during which time the testosterone stimulation occurred. After a 28-day wash-out phase the subjects received at first a 5-day cyproterone acetate monotherapy (3 × 50 mg/day orally), which caused a significant fall in testosterone values, which did not reach, however, the castrate level. During the subsequent additional therapy with the above mentioned dose of buserelin over seven days the testosterone stimulation was significantly weakened, with the testosterone levels reaching only the pre-therapeutic range. By this combined therapy the castrate level for serum testosterone was reached after no more than nine days, i. e., two weeks in advance as compared to the buserelin monotherapy. The proof has thus been established that a pre-medication of cyproterone acetate over a couple of days will suppress the testosterone stimulation phase in a subsequent therapy with LH-RH agonists thus preventing the possible clinical effects of a cancer proliferation.

Another effect of the combined therapy can be derived from the aforementioned E. O. R. T. C. study at a moment when clinical reference data are not yet available. The frequency rates for the sometimes annoying hot flushes in patients on a monotherapy with buserelin for a carcinoma of the prostate, as far as they are communicated in the literature, vary between 50 and 68 per cent. In the above study this rate could – with the additionally medicated cyproterone acetate – be reduced to 12 to 24 per cent. In the group of orchiectomized patients hot flushed occurred in 13 per cent.

Hot flushes after a bilateral orchiectomy or during an LH-RH agonist therapy are the result of the excessive fall in the peripheral androgen concentration. The attempt of a central counterregulation leads to an increased release of noradrenaline, which in turn is responsible for a disturbed thermoregulation. It has been shown in several studies that cyproterone acetate – with its centrally inhibitory antigonadotrophic component – causes a significant suppression of hot flushes in orchiectomized patients [3, 4, 11]. Whereas Claes et al. [2] suppressed also LH-RH-agonist-induced hot flushes with cyproterone acetate, this same effect was not achieved with the pure antiandrogen flutamide, which lacks an antigonadotrophic effect [10].

Clinical data of randomized studies with a long follow-up period, which might confirm the advantage of the complete androgen blockade over a castration produced by surgery or drugs alone and, consequently, back the results obtained by Labrie et al. [10] – are at present not yet available. Schroeder et al. [12] at least found identical progression rates in two seperate prospective studies with buserelin and buserelin plus cyproterone acetate, respectively.

References

[1] Boccon-Gibod, L., M. H. Laudat, M. A. Dugue et al.: Cyproterone acetate lead-in prevents initial rise of serum testosterone induced by luteinizing hormone-releasing hormone analogs in the treatment of metastatic carcinoma of the prostate. Eur. Urol. **12** (1986) 400–402.

[2] Claes, H., L. Vandenbussche, R. L. Vereecken: Treatment of advanced carcinoma of the prostate by LHRH agonists. 7. Congress Europ. Assoc. Urol., Budapest 1986, Abstr. Nr. 1016.

[3] Eaton, A. C., N. Mc Guire: Cyproterone acetate in treatment of post-orchidectomy hot flushes, double-blind cross-over trial. The Lancet **8363** (1983) 1336–1337.

[4] Gingell, J. C.: Does orchiectomy cause excessive sweating? Brit. Med. J. **288** (1984) 6418.

[5] Habenicht, U. F., E. Witthaus, F. Neumann: Antiandrogene und LH-RH-Agonisten; Endokrinologie in der Initialphase ihrer Anwendung. Akt. Urol. **17** (1986) 10–16.

[6] Hickey, D., B. Todd, M. S. Soloway: Pre-treatment testosterone levels: significance in androgen deprivation therapy. J. Urol. **136** (1986) 1038–1040.

[7] Jacobi, G. H., U. K. Wenderoth, W. Ehrenthal et al.: Endocrine and clinical evaluation of 107 patients with advanced prostatic carcinoma under long term pernasal buserelin or intramuscular decapeptyl depot treatment. In: J. G. M Klijn et al. (eds): Hormonal Manipulation of Cancer, pp. 235–248. Raven Press, New York 1987.

[8] Jacobi, G. H., U. K. Wenderoth, H. v. Wallenberg et al.: Progression and death following luteinizing hormone releasing hormone analogue monotreatment in advanced prostatic carcinoma. 82. Annual Meeting American Urological. Association Anaheim, 1987, Abstr. Nr. 609, p. 256 A.

[9] Klijn, J. G. M., H. J. De Voogt, F. H. Schröder et al.: Combined treatment with buserelin and cyproterone acetate in metastatic prostatic carcinoma. The Lancet **8453** (1985) 493.

[10] Labrie, F., A. Dupont, A. Bélanger et al.: Treatment of prostatic cancer with gonadotropin-releasing hormone agonists. Endocrine Rev. 7 (1986) 67–74.

[11] Moon, T. D.: Cyproterone acetate for treatment of hot flashes after orchiectomy. J. Urol. **134** (1985) 155–156.

[12] Schroeder, F. H., M. T. W. T. Lock, R. Chadha Dev et al.: Metastatic cancer of the prostate managed by Buserelin (HOE 766) versus Buserelin plus Cyproterone acetate (CPA). J. Urol. (1988) in Druck.

[13] Svensson, M., E. Varenhorst, B. Kagedal: Initial administration of cyproterone acetate (CPA) to prevent the rise of testosterone concentration during treatment with an LH-RH agonist in prostatic cancer. Anticancer Research 6 (1986) 379.

[14] Urwin, G. H., J. L. Williams, J. A. Kanis: Antiandrogens attenuate testosterone "flare" following zoladex depot LHRH analogue in patients with prostatic cancer. 7. Congress Europ. Assoc. Urol., Budapest 1986, Abstr. Nr. 216.

[15] Wenderoth, U. K., G. H. Jacobi: Langzeitergebnisse mit dem Gn-Rh-Analogon Buserelin (Suprefact®) bei der Behandlung des fortgeschrittenen Prostatakarzinoms seit 1981. Akt. Urol. 16 (1985) 58–63.

List of first-mentioned contributors

Prof. Dr. H. Becker, Urologische Abteilung, Marienkrankenhaus, Alfredstr. 9, D-2000 Hamburg 76

Prof. Dr. Nicholas Bruchovsky, Department of Cancer Endocrinology, Cancer Control Agency of British Columbia, 600 West 10th Avenue, Vancouver, B. C., Canada V5Z 4E6

Prof. Dr. I. Huhtaniemi, Department of Physiology, University of Turku, SF-20520 Turku 52

Prof. Dr. G. H. Jacobi, Klinikum der Johannes Gutenberg-Universität, Urologische Klinik und Poliklinik, Postfach 3960, D-6500 Mainz

Prof. Dr. D. Kirchheim, 5213 Klahanie CT, N. W., Olympia, Washington 98502, USA

Prof. Dr. F. Neumann, HD Klinische Forschung III, Schering AG, Müllerstr. 170 – 178, D-1000 Berlin 65

Dr. U. Otto, Urologische Klinik und Poliklinik, Universitäts-Krankenhaus Eppendorf, Martinistr. 52, D-2000 Hamburg 20

Prof. Dr. F. H. Schröder, Institut Urologie, Erasmus Universiteit Rotterdam, Postbus 1738, NL-300 DR Rotterdam

Prof. Franco Di Silverio, Patologia Urologica, Università di Roma, Via Feronia 146, I-00161 Roma

Dr. G. J. van Steenbrugge, Dept. Urology, Lab. Exp. Surgery, Erasmus Universiteit Rotterdam, Postbus 1738, NL-300 DR Rotterdam

Prof. Dr. U. W. Tunn, Urologische Klinik der Städt. Kliniken Offenbach, Postfach 101964, D-6050 Offenbach am Main

Dr. A. O. Turkes, Tenovus Institute for Cancer Research, University of Wales, College of Medicine, Heath Park, Cardiff, CF4 4XX Wales, UK

Dr. Eberhard Varenhorst, Chirurgische Klinik, Urologische Abteilung, Zentralkrankenhaus, S-60182 Norrköping

Prof. Dr. K. D. Voigt, Abteilung für Klin. Chemie, II. Medizinische Klinik, Universitäts-Krankenhaus Eppendorf, Martinistr. 52, D-2000 Hamburg 20

FSC
www.fsc.org
MIX
Papier | Fördert gute Waldnutzung
FSC® C083411

Zeitfracht Medien GmbH
Ferdinand-Jühlke-Straße 7
99095 Erfurt, Deutschland
produktsicherheit@kolibri360.de